AGING
PATIENTS

Mary W. Falconer, R.N., M.A., draws on extended experience in both nursing service administration and nursing education, having served most recently as instructor in pharmacology at O'Connor Hospital School of Nursing, in San Jose, California. She is the author of several widely known books, among them *The Drug, the Nurse, the Patient.*

Michael V. Altamura, M.D., Diplomate American Board of Family Practice, is clinical assistant professor, Family and Community Medicine, Stanford University Medical School. Dr. Altamura is a family physician as well, with a wide practice in geriatric medicine, and also conducts courses for paraprofessionals in the care of the aging patient.

Helen Duncan Behnke, R.N., M.A., whose professional background ranges from instructor to director of nursing education, was also senior editor, *RN Magazine*, and associate editor, *American Journal of Nursing*. Her publications, in addition to numerous articles, include *Duncan's Dictionary for Nurses* and *Guidelines for Comprehensive Nursing Care in Cancer* (as editor), both published by Springer.

AGING PATIENTS

A Guide for Their Care

Mary W. Falconer
Michael V. Altamura
Helen Duncan Behnke

Springer Publishing Company / New York

Copyright © 1976 by Springer Publishing Company, Inc.

Springer Publishing Company, Inc.
200 Park Avenue South
New York, N.Y. 10003

76 77 78 79 80 / 10 9 8 7 6 5 4 3 2 1

Library of Congress Cataloging in Publication Data

Falconer, Mary W
     Aging patients.

     Bibliography: p.
     Includes index.
     1. Geriatrics. 2. Geriatric nursing. 3. Aging.
I. Altamura, Michael V., joint author. II. Behnke,
Helen Duncan, joint author. III. Title. [DNLM:
1. Geriatric nursing. WY152 F183a]
RC952.5.F34   618.9'7   76-26943
ISBN 0-8261-1970-0
ISBN 0-8261-1971-9 pbk.

Printed in the United States of America

Contents

Preface

This book was written as a result of two of the authors' work with elderly patients, both in various institutions and in patients' homes. They had long felt the need for a handbook that could be used as a quick reference by all who care for the aged, since most of the available books seemed to have been written primarily for physicians. The actual writing was begun after Michael Altamura taught a class in gerontology to a group of paraprofessionals who were involved with the care of the aged. When asked for ways to improve the course, the students unanimously expressed a desire for a concise handbook that would help them to understand the class lectures and that could also be used later as a reference in their work. Consequently, a mimeographed outline of the course was prepared, used in further classes, revised, and finally became the manuscript for this book.

The book is designed for all paramedical personnel who are involved in the care of the aging—professional nurses, licensed practical nurses, nurses' aides, social workers, physical and occupational therapists. We also hope that the content will be of interest to people who are involved in efforts to provide a better life for the elderly.

Certain topics have been omitted, either because they were outside the scope of the book or because there are books available that adequately cover these subjects. Rehabilitation and the economic problems of the aging are two such topics. The emphasis in this book is on the common physical and mental diseases and disorders of older people, the observations that need to be made in order to correct or arrest the progress of the so-called degenerative diseases, and the actions that can be taken by professionals, paraprofessionals, and communities to help our older citizens to regain and keep their health.

Introduction

The old have always been with us. Why, then, are we currently so concerned about the problems of the aging? Among the many answers that might be given, two seem particularly important.

First, there are more older people today than there were in the past, because people are living longer. During the Greco-Roman period of history, one could expect to live about 20 years; during the Saxon-Norman period in England, life expectancy was 30 to 32 years; in the mid-nineteenth century in the United States it was 39 years; and by 1970 Americans had an average life span of 70.8 years. In 1900 only 4.1 percent of the population of this country was over 65 years of age. By 1950 this had risen to 8.2 percent and it is estimated that by 1980 14.4 percent of the population will be 65 or more years old.

Why are we living longer? Most of us enjoy better health than our ancestors did, because living conditions have improved as a result of advances in such areas as nutrition and sanitation. Also, we now have the means of preventing or curing many of the diseases that in the past were fatal to infants and young children. The second reason why the problems of the elderly are important today is that our society has changed from a farming to an industrial, technological, and urban orientation.

MAJOR PROBLEMS OF THE ELDERLY

Each aging individual has his own particular problems. Most of these problems, however, fall into the following categories.

Economic problems include those associated with food, clothing, and housing. These problems have received much attention, and since the principal emphasis in this book is on health care for the elderly, we will touch only lightly upon their economic problems.

Social problems of the elderly are closely related to their economic situation. The ever recurring question, "What is the place of the older person in our society?" has not been satisfactorily answered. As a nation we idealize youth and, to a large degree, disregard older people.

Psychological and emotional problems are often severe in the elderly. This area, too, is discussed briefly in the first section of the book.

Physical problems of the aging include more of the so-called degenerative diseases than was true in the past. This, of course, is the result of our success in preventing and curing diseases that were formerly common, and fatal, among young people. Much of the ongoing study and research in geriatrics today is devoted to finding ways of avoiding the development of the degenerative conditions that are dealt with in Section II of this book.

AGING
PATIENTS

SECTION I | The Process and Problems of Aging

What causes people to grow old? Why do some age early, chronologically, and others quite late? No one knows the answers to these questions, although there are many theories on the subject. One idea is that we are "programmed" to grow old. Other factors in aging include the following:

- *Heredity.* Members of some families seem to live longer than the average person, even though, individually, they may spend most of their lives in very different environments.
- *Environment.* In certain areas of the world people have a longer than average life span. It is interesting that studies of such areas show only a few common denominators that lead to a longer life: (1) people live most of their lives out of doors, because agriculture is the chief occupation; (2) people work hard from childhood to old age; (3) old age is a respected time of life. Such factors as smog, cigarette smoking, and the excessive use of alcohol appear to contribute to early aging and increased mortality rates.
- *Nutrition.* Good nutrition throughout life tends to delay the aging process and lengthen the life span.
- *Cosmic rays.* Constant exposure to cosmic rays may trigger the onset of aging. Some individuals are more susceptible to these rays, as well as to x-rays, than others.
- *Individual characteristics.* Obesity that results from habitual overeating can certainly speed up the aging process. Overindulgence in tobacco, alcohol, and drugs also tends to shorten the life span.

1

- *Cross linkages and cell replication* (replacement). There is evidence that cell proteins form cross linkages within the cells, causing disturbances in the physiology of the cell. The older a person becomes, the more protein cross linkages his cells have. Some cells do not replicate at all. Others replicate a given number of times and then die. Is this an inevitable process, or is it possible that cell replication can be increased in some way?

CHANGES CAUSED BY THE AGING PROCESS

Although aging is a very complex process and not completely understood, we know about many of the changes that occur, whether or not they are obvious to the aging individual or to observers.

OBSERVABLE CHANGES

Skin and Hair Changes

Dryness, inelasticity, wrinkling, and laxness of the skin are noticeable changes that occur in people as they grow old. Increasingly, lentigo (pigmented spots resembling freckles) occurs, particularly on exposed areas. Also, older people sweat less than younger people because their subcutaneous tissues contain less fluid. Body and head hair may be partly or completely lost; the hair coarsens and becomes gray or white due to loss of pigment.

Mouth and Dental Changes

The gums are more apt to be diseased than the teeth, although by the time one reaches old age one may have few, if any, teeth left. Dentures that replace lost teeth often do not fit well after years of use, and the irritation that this causes may also be a source of gum problems.

Changes in the Sense Organs

Hearing, especially for high tones, usually diminishes as one grows older, due either to fusion of the bones of the middle ear or to deterioration of the auditory nerve. Older people who do not hear everything that is said in their presence are apt to misunderstand and respond inappropriately. They often become confused and suspicious because of this.

Sight also diminishes with age, particularly for reading or close work; eyeglasses are often required for these activities around fifty years of age, and one's eyes adjust more slowly to light and dark. Cataracts and glaucoma are fairly common in older people. Diabetes mellitus may be the cause of blindness in some cases.

Changes that occur in the organs involved in smelling and tasting result in a lessening of these sensations, smell being affected more than taste.

One's sense of balance may be lost, for various reasons; a common cause is sclerosis (hardening) of the semicircular canals in the inner ear. If this loss is accompanied by vertigo (dizziness) or fainting, a careful check must be made to rule out illness or drugs as a possible cause.

Skeletomuscular Changes

Some changes that occur in the joints of the older person are evident—osteoarthritis and other arthritic conditions, for example. Loss of height is a common occurrence; this is usually due to atrophic (wasting) changes in the discs between the vertebrae, which may also cause pressure on a nerve and result in severe pain. The bones become porous and lighter (osteoporosis) from the loss of certain substances, especially calcium.

The muscles become flabby and less powerful as a result of loss of muscle substance. Leg muscle cramps, which occur more often in women than men and in obese rather than thin individuals, can be very annoying. These cramps are usually caused by poor circulation or a low blood calcium level.

Skeletomuscular changes are largely responsible for the gradual weight loss that most individuals experience as they grow older.

SUBJECTIVE CHANGES

Cellular Change and Loss

The cells that make up the tissues and organs of the body are affected by an ongoing aging process that involves cross linkages, a low respiration period, and a phenomenon that might be called "programmed limitation." That is, some cells do not replicate—once lost, they are never replaced, and nonfunctioning tissue cells take their place. This is especially true of nerve and muscle cells, the replacement being neuroglia in the nervous system and fibrous tissue in the muscles. Even cells that do replicate have their limits; they divide a certain number of times (often as many as 40 to 50 times) and then die.

Systemic Changes

Gradually, the efficiency of the various body systems declines, resulting in breakdowns in these systems. Transmission between systems also slows down. One cause of these changes is the loss of body fluids, which tends to make the cells and tissues of the systems "brittle" and less able to function efficiently.

Cardiovascular changes occur frequently. The heart is apt to become enlarged, more often in men than in women. Blood pressure often increases, particularly the systolic pressure, and medical measures may be necessary to reduce it. However, unless the blood pressure suddenly rises to seriously high levels, it may be unwise to try to lower it, because this could deprive the brain of needed oxygen and nutrients. Chest expansion decreases and, as a consequence, the vital capacity of the lungs also decreases.

Nervous system changes are often the cause of serious problems for older people. There may be a decreased cerebral blood flow, which lowers the amount of oxygen and glucose going to the brain. This decrease is irregular and tends to block out certain areas of the brain. The electroencephalogram (the tracing of brain waves) shows a lowered level of activity in the brain. Actual loss of brain cells occurs, a process that is increased in alcohol users. Alcohol is poisonous to the brain; it has been reported that one ounce of whiskey destroys approximately 5000 brain cells.

Mental and Emotional Changes

Mental and emotional changes may be profound, or so slight as to be nonexistent. Loss of memory for recent events may be an early sign of deterioration. Depression, which is usually unconscious in young people, is conscious in the elderly. There is a decrease in one's responses to painful stimuli, and this may cause serious problems if the older person is badly injured or burned without realizing it. Confusion is common and often leads the patient to act irrationally. The circuits in the "computer" become crossed and the results are unpredictable. Ability to understand the spoken word, however, is often superior to that of younger people.

The process of aging, always slow, decreases progressively as the person grows older. However, aging is a natural process, as much a part of life as growth and development are, for we are "born to die."

SOCIAL AND PSYCHOLOGICAL PROBLEMS

In recent years better sanitation, health care, and medical services have markedly increased the life span. But this increase has been a mixed blessing, since people who now live longer do not always have the satisfactions the added years should bring. As so often occurs, science has outstripped social progress.

WHAT IS THE SOURCE OF THE PROBLEMS?

Changes in Our Society

Many of the problems of the aged come, at least in part, from the industrialization and urbanization of our society. When life in this country was largely rural, the family farm was the basic social unit and the older generation created few if any problems. The family unit often consisted of three or even four generations living under one roof, and houses were built with this in mind. Today, we wonder how these people withstood the lack of privacy, but they did not have the expectations as the present generation. Everyone, even small children, expected to work hard. Their few pleasures were cherished and enjoyed by the whole family together. They made their own entertainment and were not, as is the custom now, entertained. It was not an easy life, but it was by no means all drudgery. No one felt abused.

The picture of Grandma or Aunt Celia sitting in a rocking chair knitting seems to us today to be a complete waste of time. Actually, they were making the socks, mittens, scarves, and sweaters that were essential for the family. Knitting was not the only task older women performed. They helped prepare the food for cooking or preserving; did some or all of the cooking; churned the butter; made the soap; washed, carded, and spun the wool, flax, or cotton for clothes; and often wove the cloth as well. Interestingly, the word "spinster," meaning "old maid," came from the fact that the older unmarried female member of the household usually did the spinning.

The older man in the family was usually the head of the entire establishment. He might not engage in hard physical work, but he saw that it was done. He helped with the chores, fed the livestock, gardened, and cleaned and repaired the farm tools and equipment. He was also often the "handyman" around the house.

High on the almost limitless list of tasks performed by older people in the past was baby-sitting. This function rarely involved sitting, however, for the grandparents were often the ones who taught children many skills and helped teach them a moral outlook on life. This is a privilege denied most children today.

Retirement

Another problem of the aged is caused by the fact that industry and government have set 65 as the age at which an individual becomes old and incapable of working. In addition, government, in its social security regulations, has said that one may not work, except in a very limited way, between the ages of 65 and 72, but that after 72 one can work and earn as much as one likes. Thus, many years that could have been productive are spent in idleness and often unhappiness because of the feeling that one has been put "on the shelf." Of course, it is well known that one person may be unemployable at 35, whereas another may still be a productive worker at 75; some standards need to be set, but do they need to be so inflexible? The medical and health sciences foresee a life span of 100 years in the future. If retirement from useful employment is set at 60, which seems to be the present trend, what will the individual do with the 40 years of life that he will spend as an "old" person? Why is the younger person so much more important than the older one today? Because our society idealizes youth. In an age when discrimination against minority groups is considered intolerable, the bias against the old is often overlooked.

HOW DO OLDER PEOPLE VIEW THEIR PROBLEMS?

If all the problems of the aged could be expressed in one word, that word would be "fear"—fear of dependence, of financial need, of being misunderstood, of being considered "in the way," of being useless, of crippling illness, and of death.

The fear of illness is not confined to the older age group, but it is more pronounced. Older people realize that they are at an age when sickness is more apt to occur and that many of the diseases of the elderly are crippling and incapacitating.

Fear of financial dependence is tied to the decision about where one will live. The extent of this problem is staggering. Hundreds of thousands of elderly people live (or exist) in so-called nursing homes. Others eke out a lonely existence in hotel rooms or small apartments. Many others live unhappily with relatives who, though well intentioned, find the older person a burden. Today's houses are built for one family only; there is no room for relatives. Also, it has become customary for each person, even an infant, to have his own room.

WHERE SHALL THE OLDER PERSON LIVE?

Of the many factors to be considered in deciding where the older person should live, three are of prime importance: (1) Is the individual a single person or is there a spouse or relative? (2) What is the individual's financial status? (3) What is the individual's mental and physical condition?

The usual choices of where one should live are: with relatives or alone; in a house, a mobile home, an apartment, or a single room (usually in a hotel or boarding house); in a retirement village; or in a nursing home. Living with relatives has the advantage of being close to those one cares most about, although it is well known that "familiarity breeds contempt." Another advantage is that the younger members of the family can watch out and care for the older members. If the older person is financially independent, his contribution can be a real help to the young family. But if both parents are financially dependent, and must live with their children, the added cost of their maintenance can be a real drain on the family budget. When it is decided that an older person shall live with a young family, a few rules will help keep things running smoothly:

1. Plan for the older person to have a room of his own to which he can retire whenever he wishes.
2. Be frank with each other.
3. Discuss any grievances openly in the family group.
4. Do not quarrel about child rearing. Everyone should understand from the beginning who is the final authority in regard to disciplining the children.

5. Do not ignore the frustrations of the older person and do not hurry him to do things and to come to decisions.
6. Treat the damages of a long life with tenderness.
7. If the older person is physically able, let him do certain chores and give him time to do them.

If the older person has a satisfactory home and is financially able to keep it up, this is probably the best place for him. Home is where he is used to being; it is familiar. The older one gets, the more one dislikes change. A home gives a person something to do—a yard to care for, housekeeping chores to do, meals to cook, and so on. If cooking becomes too much of a burden, "meals on wheels" are obtainable in many communities. If friends or relatives live nearby, so much the better. Often younger relatives are overprotective and fearful that the older person will have an accident. However, many older individuals would rather risk an accident than to move into a more sheltered and dependent situation.

Of course there should be some means of checking on older people who live alone. For those who have no relatives or immediate friends who can telephone every day, many communities have volunteer groups whose members telephone daily to see if things are all right. If not, a volunteer will investigate or send the proper people to do so.

What has just been said about living in one's own house may also be said about living in an apartment. Apartment living has some advantages as well as some disadvantages not found in one's own house. One advantage is that an apartment building usually has a caretaker who is available in case of need. Another is that the apartment dweller often becomes friendly with others living in the same building, and this not only brightens his outlook but may be a source of help in time of emergency. One disadvantage is that an apartment is more confining than a house—there is no lawn to mow, no garden to care for. Children living in the building can also be a disadvantage.

Living alone in a single room is even more confining than an apartment. If a person has a room and board arrangement, he may receive a more balanced diet than he would if he tried to prepare his food in his room or ate in restaurants. Some older people deteriorate rapidly when living alone in one room; others live that way for years and keep mentally and physically fit, particularly if they have friends nearby to see and talk to.

Living in a mobile home is similar in many ways to living in a separate house, but it has its own advantages and disadvantages. Organized social and recreational activities are usually provided, and a stimulating and helpful spirit of friendship often develops. People are always available in an emergency, and neighbors tend to look out for one another. However, most mobile home courts are located away from city centers, and public transportation is often unavailable, because such places are planned for people who have automobiles and are able to drive them.

What has been said of a house and a mobile home may also be said of the retirement village. When selecting a mobile home court or retirement village, one should consider cost, location (nearness to churches, banks, shopping centers), and availability of public transportation. Are recreational facilities provided? Are medical, dental, and nursing care available? Is there a hospital nearby? Does one rent or buy the home, and must one's own furnishings be brought? If the location is far away from a previous home, are the weather and climate such that one can adjust to them?

Whether the older person should enter a nursing home is a serious question, which should be carefully studied in cooperation with the family physician. Nursing homes are a big business today, and, unlike most hospitals, are profit-making establishments. Naturally, to make a profit, they take in as many patients as possible, charge as much as they can, and provide limited services. In most cases, these homes should be used only for patients who are physically or mentally incapable of caring for themselves and who have no relative who can help them. Younger people often feel that it is a disgrace to have a member of the family in a nursing home, but sometimes there is no alternative.

The Pros and Cons of Nursing Home Living

Nursing homes, by whatever name they are called, are, in reality, mausoleums for the aged. Often three or four beds are crowded so tightly into one small room that it is necessary to move beds to get a stretcher or wheelchair in or out and patients have no place to keep personal items. There may not even be a clock in the room. Is it any wonder that patients in this kind of environment become confused and depressed? It is true, however, that many people who work in nursing homes try very hard to give their patients the best possible care. They are often young and dedicated people working against almost impossible odds.

Before deciding on a nursing home for an older person, one

should consider cost and how the bills are paid—weekly, monthly, or a lump sum for life. Do the fees include all meals, special diets, extra nourishment, laundry service? Does the nursing home provide clothing or does the resident wear his own? Are recreational, occupational, and physical activities available, and is a trained therapist in charge of these? Is the home near the person's relatives and friends? What are the visiting privileges? How many beds to a room? Does the place seem clean and well cared for? Do residents get a chance to be outside in good weather? What about medical care? Does the family physician remain in charge or does the facility employ its own doctor? Is there a registered nurse or licensed practical nurse in charge around the clock, or just in the daytime?

There will always be a need for places where the senile older person can be cared for, but the multitude of nursing homes is, in the opinion of many, evidence of a social failure. Many who have studied the problem feel that the majority of patients in these homes are there because of deterioration caused by boredom, lack of purpose in life, or lack of someone who cares about them.

What is the answer? Naturally, there is no single answer, but those who are responsible for helping to decide where the older person should live can help that person greatly by keeping the following facts in mind. Whatever the facility decided upon, it should be centrally located, near a shopping center, bank, church, library, and public transportation. As far as being in a quiet location is concerned, this is not always of primary importance, since most older people have some hearing loss and a really quiet place may be one with no sound whatever.

If possible, the building should be of the hotel or motel type, with gradations for individuals of varying abilities. The requirements should include:

1. No stairs. Ramps and elevators should be used for moving from one level to another. Fire escapes should be chutes that are ample and easily entered.
2. Doors and hallways should be wide enough to allow for wheelchairs and for moving of patients or furniture if necessary.
3. Small apartments should be provided for couples and single persons able to use them.
4. All rooms should be single occupancy. They should be provided with a bath, a large closet and other storage space, and a telephone.

5. A central kitchen and dining room with tray service for those who require it.
6. A dietician should be in charge of the food service, and special diets should be available for those who need them.
7. For those who are ill or are likely to become ill, the rooms should be equipped with closed-circuit television and monitoring services with a central station manned 24 hours a day by a competent nurse.
8. All rooms and apartments should be equipped with a two-way talking system connected with the central station.
9. Medical, dental, and nursing services should be available. A well-equipped examining room should be provided for such services.
10. There should be a large lobby or parlor on the main floor with smaller rooms off it where visitors can talk with their relatives or friends without interruption.
11. A hobby or crafts room, with a part-time occupational therapist in charge, is a must. Volunteers can help out in this activity when the therapist is not available.
12. An infirmary or hospital should be available nearby for the acutely ill.
13. Routines should be flexible: One of the criticisms of nursing homes is that all patients must conform to a routine that is set for the convenience of the personnel. Often this is not explained to the new patient. Imagine a person who is used to getting up at 8:00, having his meals at 8:30, 1:00, and 7:00, and going to bed at 10:00 or 11:00, suddenly having to get up at 6:00, having his meals at 6:30, 11:00, and 5:00, and having to go to bed at 9:00!

HOW TO MAKE THE LATER YEARS COUNT

Attitudes toward the elderly and terms used to express these attitudes may be neutral, positive, or negative. "Old," "old age," and "the aged" are rather neutral terms used to imply simply that the person referred to has passed the period of life known as middle age. Positive terms are "elderly" and "venerable," the latter usually being reserved for persons of distinction in some capacity. "Aging" is another positive term that implies an ongoing process but does not put all people past middle age in one group regardless of their physical and mental status. Negative terms include "superannuated" and "senile." The term "superannuated" usually implies that the person can no longer fulfill the functions of the position or status he once held. "Senile" may mean that the person has deteriorated physically, but is more often used to indicate loss of mental ability, with or without physical deterioration. Sometimes, with energy, patience, and a long period of rehabilitation, senility can be reversed, but of course it is better to prevent it if possible. Medical advances have provided ways to minimize the effects and development of certain degenerative conditions, and these should be utilized. In addition, a regimen of life that will delay the onset of these conditions will pay rich rewards in the form of a healthier, more constructive, and more enjoyable life for the elderly.

CLOSE THE GENERATION GAP

We often speak of the "generation gap"; perhaps a better expression would be the "technological gap." In reality, the population is a continuum, with no beginning, no end, and no gaps. The fantastic technological and scientific advances of the twentieth century, however, have created a gap between the young, who take the modern world for granted and speak its language, and the elderly, many of whom do not understand the changes that have occurred during their lifetimes.

To realize how older people feel, just imagine the world as it was in 1900. The horseless carriage was one of the wonders of the world. There were no airplanes, radios, television, no man-made fission or fusion, no computers, only a few telephones, some gaslights, and a few electric lights. Most labor-saving household appliances did not exist.

It is almost impossible for the youth of today to imagine such a world; it is equally hard for older people to appreciate fully the feelings of those who have known only our scientifically and technologically advanced society. Many older people have seen the change from gas lamps to neon lights, horse and carriage to jet planes, from multigenerational homes to the two-generational family. Is it any wonder that many are confused?

Older people tend to live in the past; the older they get, the greater is their tendency to do so. Such clinging to a dead world is distasteful to a young person. Moreover, the young person is impatient with the slowness of the older generation, its failure to adjust to today's pace.

Several other basic differences between the age groups cause conflict and misunderstanding:

- Youth is in a hurry—whatever takes a long time to accomplish is not finished or even started. In contrast, the older person works slowly and deliberately, and does not mind attempting something that may take a long time.
- Many young people have a great store of knowledge, but lack understanding; many older people have much less knowledge, but more experience, wisdom, and understanding.
- A young person is healthy and able to do a lot of work in a given period of time. Most older people, on the other hand, have some physical disorder or handicap; they may be able to do the same work, but it takes longer.
- A young person thinks in the present; old people are apt to think in the past. Neither are too likely to think in the future.
- The elderly tend to have a narrow vision, sometimes too narrow. They elaborate details; small things are important to them. Young people, on the other hand, "think big." Older peoples' experience often shows how futile these big ideas are.
- The language of the two groups often differs greatly. Young people use such terms as "input," "aerodynamics," "cassette," and so on. Many older people do not understand the real meaning of these terms any more than young people understand "horse-and-buggy" language.
- Each group feels superior to the other and looks down upon the other.
- Young people tend to shun older people. Possibly they see themselves as old and they do not like it.
- Cultural differences make the young person sometimes fear contact with older individuals.
- Many older individuals (not necessarily just those over 65) feel that the young people of today do not show them proper respect. This is sometimes true, but for understandable reasons. Often the most critical older person does not deserve the respect he desires. There are many older people, however, who do deserve respect.

DOS AND DON'TS FOR THOSE WHO
CARE FOR THE ELDERLY

Before specifying how young people can better relate to and care for the elderly, it might be useful to do away with some common misconceptions, such as "old age makes people different"; "old people expect too much"; "grandparents want to be with their grandchildren all the time." In truth, older people have the same needs as everyone else. Most of them want independence, status, health, a chance to be useful, someone who cares about them and is kind and patient with them. They want to be able to help when others need it; in fact, they much prefer to be able to do for others than to have others do for them. They want to make their own decisions. They want economic security. They want pleasant family relationships, but that does not necessarily mean that they want to live with the family. Some are very mature, while others are quite immature. Some have dual personalities such as the adolescent often has—at times independent, at times almost as dependent as a young child.

Younger persons who care for the elderly (nurses, relatives, friends) will find it helpful to cultivate thoughtfulness, tolerance, patience, tact, interest, friendliness, persuasiveness, flexibility, and understanding; and to avoid pity, condescension, and impatience. The following suggestions will help to improve communication with older patients.

Often younger people do not realize that failing hearing or eyesight are the main causes of introversion and loss of contact with reality. When speaking to an older person, face him; call him by name and state your own name; speak slowly, clearly, and with good enunciation—do not shout. Most older people have some hearing loss, but a loud voice does not make understanding easier. Background noise is very annoying for the hard-of-hearing, whether old or not, so try to eliminate as much background noise as possible before trying to converse with hard-of-hearing individuals. If the person does not seem to understand what you are saying, try again, rewording the sentence; he may not recognize the words you are using. If his answer seems inappropriate, he may not have heard correctly because of some physical disturbance of the ear or brain, but he may think he has heard and answered properly. When what is being said to him is important, it may be necessary to use some other form of expression, such as writing. Never whisper in the presence of a hard-of-hearing person or speak to others in a tone he cannot hear; this makes him suspicious and defensive. If the person also has poor vision, place your hand lightly on his hand or wrist while you speak; the vibrations created by your voice will help him to understand what is being said. It may be helpful for him to be fitted with a hearing aid.

To help the older person overcome the effects of failing eyesight, use fairly bright colors in the rooms the person uses, and make sure that lines of demarcation (for example, around doorways) are clearly indicated. If bright colors are not suitable, soft greens, rose, or cream are better than pure white, which reflects light well and may make seeing difficult for some people. The same may be said of high-gloss enamels and highly polished woodwork or furniture. Gray, blue, and dark colors are depressing; bright orange and red are stimulating and are thought to increase hostility and aggressiveness. All written material should be printed in large type. Most public libraries offer excellent materials in large type—books and periodicals. In one instance, a patient was accused of not following the diet her physician had prescribed. An alert nurse discovered that the directions were printed in type too small for the patient to read; when given to her in type large enough for her to see she followed the directions accurately. Typed material is usually better than hand-written material.

Remember that older people think and react slowly. A person who has suffered any brain damage is likely to react slowly and in a confused manner. To avoid confusion, consider some of the things (in addition to brain damage) that may cause it—change of routine, change of environment, meeting new people, seeing someone after a long separation, loss or separation from a loved one, the onset of illness, stress situations of any kind. The list is almost endless. There are many little things one can do to help prevent the older person from becoming disoriented. Place a clock with a luminous dial and large numbers in the room, and a calendar with large numbers. The person's name should be printed in large letters on the door or on the bed if he occupies a room with others (particularly if he has poor vision, since this is often accompanied by disorientation). When you greet a person in the morning, say something like "This is Friday, March 12th," and if it is a holiday, birthday, or other special day, mention that.

Always call the patient by name, but avoid using first names as well as such terms as "grandpa," "grannie," or "nana." Be particularly careful to address women as "Miss" or "Mrs." Otherwise, you may bring up very unpleasant memories to someone whose only grandchild is dead, someone who has never married, or someone who never had any children, much less grandchildren, and this has been her unfulfilled life's dream. When visiting an older person, introduce yourself; if you have married since the person last saw you, mention the name by which he knew you and recall some incident he may remember. It is painfully embarrassing for an older person not to recognize someone he should know. If a patient who has been well oriented suddenly becomes confused for no apparent reason, he should have a physical checkup, since confusion often is a sign of the onset of an acute illness such as pneumonia.

Confusion and disorientation often result when an individual first enters a nursing home, because everything that has been familiar to him is suddenly gone. This reaction is especially noticeable if he is put into a room with two, three, or more patients, some of whom are senile. The individual may take to hoarding, may become mute and appear to be actually psychotic, or may become angry and vent his resentment on the staff. Suspicion may lead to apparent paranoia, when in fact the individual is just trying to assert himself and maintain his self-image. It should be remembered too that often the patient brings with him the customs of another time and sometimes of another country; he cannot be expected to change them overnight.

Younger people who care for the elderly sometimes fail to recognize that the newly admitted patient, who is expected to conform unquestioningly to a routine that is entirely different from the one he is long accustomed to, may become confused and disoriented. Careful explanation of routines and regulations, repeated as often as necessary, will help to prevent many problems of adjustment.

The physical environment of the older person needs special attention. Many older people have circulatory difficulties and, like infants, need a warm and even temperature. The usual day temperature in their rooms should not drop below 72° or the night temperature below 65°. Higher temperatures may be required in certain cases. Hallways should also be kept warm at all times, because many older patients must go to the bathroom during the night. Ventilation should be indirect; that is, direct flow of air on the patient should be avoided.

Even though the elderly are usually hard of hearing, loud noises should be avoided, especially at night. Attendants often forget this and make many unnecessary and sometimes sudden loud noises. The same is true for light—too bright a light or one that is directly in the patient's eyes is disturbing to anyone trying to sleep. However, a night light strong enough to show furniture and doorways is essential for the older person who must get up at night.

The older patient often complains of insomnia. When he says "I didn't sleep a wink last night," it may be more imagination than truth. However, arguing with the patient about his sleep will only antagonize him uselessly. If possible, check the amount of sleep he actually gets, and, if it is found to be insufficient, notify the physician.

If the patient needs surgery or special treatment, but is reluctant to have it done, let him express his fears. Be a good listener. Explain, if you can, what is to be done, why, and the probable results. If you are not able to do this, talk to the physician or surgeon about it and ask him to explain it to the patient or to you. He has probably already told the patient, but often the patient has not understood what he has said. Repeated explanations of what seems obvious to the nurse or attendant are often needed.

If the patient is irritable and difficult to deal with, let him "blow off steam." He may be protesting the confinement, trying to assert his independence. Try to find the cause of his behavior. Possibly he has painful arthritis; perhaps someone promised to visit him and failed to do so; he may have been promised a trip outside the institution and the person who was to take him did not appear. Of course, it may also be the sign of an oncoming illness.

Do not do for the elderly what they can do for themselves. Much irritability and resentment is brought about by the young attendant taking over and doing rapidly what the older person could have done at a more leisurely pace. The patient thinks he is not doing things right or as well as others think he should, and this is degrading. Confinement in a nursing home often makes an individual feel useless, worthless, neglected, and abandoned. The family may have feelings of guilt which are sensed by the older person, who may misinterpret them. Then there are those, both patients and their families, who expect the doctor and the staff to work miracles. The patient may not realize that his confinement is final; he expects to get well and go home. If and when he realizes the finality of the situation, the shock may be severe.

Most importantly, the patient should not be allowed to remain in bed. Get him up into a chair or wheelchair as often as possible. Have him walk if he is able and get outside whenever weather and other circumstances permit. Walking and a change of scenery often prevent or alleviate increasing dependence, incontinence, irritability, depression, and confusion. It also delays the onset of senility and keeps the patient from withdrawing from society and from life. Reasonable precautions should be taken to prevent accidents, of course, but to shelter the older person from all possible accidents is to shelter him from life. (See Appendix C, Evaluation of Activities of Daily Living.)

MAINTAIN A POSITIVE HEALTH PROGRAM

Good health habits for the elderly include regular and adequate elimination of body wastes; regular bathing and care of hair and nails; regular dental check-ups, whether or not one wears dentures; and regular physical examinations.

Moderation in all things is a good rule for the aging to follow. If one is a smoker, it may not be wise to abruptly quit the habit, but smoking can and should be limited. The same holds for the use of alcohol and self-prescribed drugs.

An older person who has enjoyed his career should be allowed to continue working as long as he is physically and mentally able to do so, either part-time or full-time, as the situation allows. Whether or not he needs the income is beside the point. However, a boring job is not good for one's health, and no job at all can quickly lead to senility, particularly in persons who have had a very active working life during their younger years.

The aging person should try to avoid stress—physical, emotional, and psychological. Stress releases the emergency hormones in the body, leads to high blood pressure, and may lead to a heart attack or stroke. If one has a tendency to become tense, one should learn to relax, to "let down" physically and mentally until one regains his calm and healthy outlook, but relaxation should not be carried so far that one loses all incentive and drive, for this leads to introversion and regression.

It may be hard for the older person who lives alone to provide an adequate diet for himself. In many communities there are now places where persons can go to receive free or low-cost meals at least once a day. Also, the "meals on wheels" arrangement in many areas makes it possible for the shut-in to have well-balanced meals delivered to a home at minimum cost. The food may not be what one would select for oneself if one were able to do so, but the meals planned by community agencies usually contain the food elements needed to maintain adequate nourishment.

Regular exercise that is suited to the individual's needs, desires, and abilities is essential. The important point about exercise is that it should be engaged in regularly. Gardening, walking, housework, and crafts all give one some exercise. Certain outdoor activities such as jogging should only be done with the physician's permission, but, if one is reasonably healthy, this can usually be obtained. (See Appendixes D, E, and F.)

Recreation should be part of every aging person's health program, whether he is in an institution or at home. The possibilities for engaging in recreational activities are many and varied. Those who work with the elderly can do a great deal to help develop interests and activities that make a person's later years healthy and satisfying. A good way to begin is to try to find out what the individual's past preferences and interests were and what his present abilities will permit him to do. The patient's family and friends, the social worker, church personnel, former co-workers, and fellow club members are all sources of information. The information should focus on the person's past abilities and strengths, not his disabilities and weaknesses. How has he used his free time since retirement—passively or actively? How did he use his free time during his younger years? If he enjoyed some activity that is no longer available to him or impossible for him to engage in, can some less active activity be substituted? Would he work best with a large group, a small one, or alone? What community resources are available for helping him reenter or retain contact with the world around him?

All nursing homes should have some kind of recreation program. Television and radio are almost always available, but it is not desirable that the patient become dependent on this type of entertainment; it can and does lead to introversion in many older people. Outside groups—high school or college students, especially drama, music, and dance majors, Girl Scouts, and church groups—are often more than willing to come in and entertain patients, and the response they get is very rewarding. Weekly visits by an occupational therapist can introduce many activities that can be carried on in her absence, with the help of volunteers. All patients who are physically able should be encouraged to take part in some activity and should be allowed to choose what they wish to do. A good leader will help create self-confidence and promote self-expression in patients. Some simple activities that all can enjoy are games, puzzles, and parties (celebrating holidays, birthdays, and so on).

BUILD POSITIVE MENTAL HEALTH
THROUGH SOCIALIZATION

In institutions for the elderly it is fairly easy to organize groups of patients with similar interests and talents. An occupational therapist is the ideal person to start such groups, and volunteers can carry on during her absence if she is a part-time employee.

Socialization centers are available in many cities. They are staffed by professional social workers, occupational therapists, public health nurses, and volunteers. They are designed to keep borderline senile patients from regressing further, and to restore contact with life for many. Very often the effect on the individual who takes part in such a program is the arrest of further deterioration and even the achievement of a higher level of mental activity. These centers usually accept a very limited number of patients (ten to fifteen) and operate five days a week. The patients, most of whom live alone, are transported to the center by bus or cars, and spend most of the day there. Those able to pay are charged a small fee for luncheon. Activities vary with the group and their abilities. The men often do carpentry, metal work, or photography. Women patients often knit, sew, crochet, or do some form of art work. The group should be kept small and as nearly intact as possible so that the patient does not have to continually adjust to different people.

An aid to socialization known as "reality orientation" is often used. The leader of the group may begin by asking: "What day of the week is it?" "What is the date?" "What month is it?" "What year is it?" "What kind of weather are we having today?" "Where are we?" "What did we do yesterday?" The answers can be printed in large letters on a blackboard. Of course, this procedure could also be followed in the patient's home or in a nursing home.

For older persons who are still mentally active and in touch with their environment, retired persons' clubs or senior citizens' clubs are excellent sources of contact with people of similar age and interests. Often these clubs are sponsored by churches, but most are nonsectarian and offer companionship with people of many differing backgrounds. They usually provide a variety of programs to suit varied tastes and interests, and offer counseling services as well. Classes in art, sewing, and handiwork of various kinds may be offered and sometimes members are able to teach others the skills that they know, which is good for both teacher and pupil. Some of the centers serve one or more meals a day at a minimum cost (or for free to those who cannot pay), thus assuring an adequate diet for those who live in single rooms or alone in apartments.

If there is no senior citizens' club in the immediate area, or if programs of those already established are not of interest, a new club can be started by bringing together a few people who are interested in similar activities. For example, clubs have been formed by people who enjoy such activities as giving and hearing book reviews; discussing any topic such as art, drama, music, flowers, political issues; playing cards and other games; debating; creative writing; collecting stamps, coins, or other objects. However, one does not need to belong to a club to enjoy many pleasurable creative activities alone (or perhaps with another person), such as carpentry, furniture refinishing, redecorating one's home, making jewelry, collecting rocks, making rugs, needlework, block printing, weaving, and so on.

Many of these activities can be profitable, but the main thing is to get the older person interested in some activity that will take his thoughts from himself. Depression and regression set in as soon as one begins to think only of one's own aches, pains, and troubles. This does not mean that illness (physical or emotional) should be ignored. Regular examinations by a physician, ophthalmologist, or dentist should be a yearly event. When care by a specialist has been recommended and treatment instituted to eliminate remediable conditions, the matter should no longer be worried about. Worry can lead to anxiety and depression. "Do not build bridges when there is only a mud puddle to cross" is a healthful saying for the older person to keep in mind.

Rehabilitation programs are sometimes very helpful in overcoming or reversing the effects of some disorders of the elderly. In some communities these programs are accomplishing a great deal, but often they are planned by enthusiastic, dedicated young people without the knowledge or cooperation of those most concerned—the elderly themselves. Perhaps the term "rehabilitation" should be reserved for efforts to help those who have physical limitations resulting from an injury or disabling illness rather than from advancing age. We might better think of regaining or restoring the abilities and faculties that have been altered as a result of the aging process.

BUILD POSITIVE PERSPECTIVES ON DYING, DEATH, AND BEREAVEMENT

It is impossible to work with elderly people for any length of time without coming face to face with dying, death, and bereavement. Professional and paraprofessional people need to come to grips with their own feelings and philosophy about death as well as to understand their patients' feelings on this subject.

People vary greatly in their attitudes toward death and their ideas of life after death. Some believe in an afterlife in which the good are rewarded and the evil are punished. Others believe in an afterlife in which everyone is treated alike, or in death as a step toward spiritual perfection (Nirvana), in which the individual spirit will be reincarnated as another physical being until this perfection is reached. Some view death as final for the individual but believe his spirit remains in the people he has affected during his lifetime. Still others see death as final and afterlife nonexistent.

Almost everyone views death as a release from the suffering of this world and relief from pain if they are in pain, as is often the case. Even if one does not believe in life after death, what could be better than a dreamless, uninterrupted sleep? However, most people, even those with religious faith and an intellectual perception of death as a release to a better life fear death. No one has returned from death to tell us what it is like.

Whether one does or does not fear death, the dying person needs someone to lean upon, someone who will listen and not pass judgment. Studies have shown that most patients realize when the end of life is near, yet the question frequently arises as to whether or not the patient should be told that he is dying. In the face of research that has been done, there seems to be no reason why a person should not be told, although there is no absolute answer to this question. Naturally, the attendant is not the person to make this decision, but he may be able to tell whether or not the patient suspects that death is near and report this to the physician, who, in consultation with the family, will decide if the patient should be told.

Dr. Elizabeth Kübler-Ross stated in her book *On Death and Dying* that the dying patient (and, of course, his family) pass through several stages. The first is one of disbelief: "No! Not me!" Secondly, he asks, "Why me?" At this stage the patient may be combative, wondering why the doctors and nurses are not making him well. The third stage is one of bargaining: "Yes me, but." The patient thinks of all the things he will do if he is just allowed to recover. The final stage is one of depression, followed by resignation: "Yes, me." Of course, not all patients go through all of these stages; some never reach resignation, others never experience the first stages. As always, patients differ widely, but if the attendant is aware of these changes in the patient's thinking it will help him to understand the person's moods.

Many nurses and doctors are not emotionally prepared to support the dying patient, but those who care for the elderly should make every effort to overcome any ambivalent feelings they may have about death and learn to listen to the dying person who may wish to express his fears and doubts. A religious or spiritual leader may be the best-prepared listener, but such a person may not be available at the moment the patient wishes to talk. The nurse or attendant may not want to take time to sit down and listen and talk to the patient because they have many important things to do in caring for the living, but they should never refuse to take a few minutes to comfort and listen to the dying patient.

Many institutions, hospitals as well as nursing homes, have strict rules concerning visitors, which they will not break even for the dying, inexcusable as this may seem. Almost everone has someone on whom they rely and lean, and this person at least should be allowed to be with a dying patient if they wish to be.

It is the attendant's responsibility to notify a representative of whatever church or congregation the critically ill patient belongs to, even if the nursing home or hospital has its own chaplain. This should not be left until death is near, since the patient may wish to talk to a religious advisor of his own faith as soon as he realizes that his situation is critical, and while he is still mentally alert.

Because most people now die in institutions and the bodies are taken directly to a mortuary, family contact with death is often lacking, especially if the family has not been allowed to be with the patient at the time of death. It can be quite a shock (even if one knows that it is coming) to receive a telephone call saying, "Your mother has just died. What mortuary do you want me to call?" Yet this is not an uncommon occurrence. The person making the call may be experienced in this duty, but the person receiving it may be experiencing the fact of death for the first time and may have just lost the person he loved most in the world. In the case of sudden, relatively unexpected death, the person notifying the family should make every effort to be tactful, understanding, and supportive.

Should the terminally ill patient be kept alive by artificial means, and, if so, for how long? Again, there is no universal answer to this question. Some physicians feel that life should be prolonged as long as possible by whatever means are available. However, modern science being what it is, this may mean an indefinite existence without, in many cases, any hope of recovery. If an electroencephalogram shows no brain waves, is there any point to trying to keep the other systems of the body functioning? In most cases, the physician consults with the family and does what they together think is best.

How can the physician, nurse, or attendant support the family when a loved one is dying? This is an important function of those who have taken care of the patient. Often, reassurance that all that could have been done was done will help the family to accept the death more easily. Understanding and consideration are the most important qualities at this time.

KEEP CONTACT WITH REALITY

To prevent senility and to reestablish contact with reality when it has been lost require every available resource—family, friends, clubs, churches, community agencies, and volunteer workers. Most of the activities outlined here cost little to provide, but it may take weeks or months to restore a more normal outlook on life in the regressed elderly person. Younger people who work with the aging are often impatient to see the results of their efforts, but these come about slowly and the worker must learn to be patient and persistent.

The popular saying, "You are as young as you feel" is very true. Chronological age means little at any time of life. A five-year-old may have a mental age of seven, a physical age of eight, and a social age of four. The same can be said of individuals at any age. Mental ability is often a better gauge of one's potential for healthful, productive living than physical condition or actual age in years. Everyone knows about the intellectual capacity and output of some of the world's great men in the later years of life. We cannot all be "great" but we should all be allowed and encouraged to be as great as we are capable of being during all the days of our lives.

Welfare, social security, medicare benefits, and various community programs have changed the picture for older people in many ways, some good, some not so good. Society has begun to realize that it has an obligation to its older citizens, but these benefits are a sort of "conscience money." Rather than recognizing that most older people are willing and able to care for themselves if given half a chance, our society's attitude seems to be "since you cannot work, we will try to make it up to you by giving you a handout." The fact that the "handout" is not adequate to maintain the elderly seems to be ignored.

Perhaps the most thoughtful advice one can give to those who work with the elderly including those who have some physical or mental disability, is to keep in mind the provisions of the Senior

Citizen's Charter, which was drawn up at the 1960 White House Conference on Aging:

Each of our senior citizens, regardless of race, color or creed, is entitled to:

1. The right to be useful.
2. The right to obtain employment based on merit.
3. The right to freedom from want in old age.
4. The right to a fair share of the communities' recreational, educational, and medical resources.
5. The right to obtain decent housing suited to the needs of the later years.
6. The right to the moral and financial support of one's family in so far as is consistent with the best interest of the family.
7. The right to live independently, as one chooses.
8. The right to live and die in dignity.
9. The right of access to all knowledge available on how to improve the later years of life.

Sixteen years later, how many of these rights has society granted to the elderly?

HEALTH CARE FOR THE ELDERLY

REPORTING A PATIENT'S CONDITION

Reporting a patient's condition to the physician may be as varied as there are patients, physicians, and disease conditions; therefore, no hard and fast rules can be set up. However, certain general procedures are recognized.

1. When reporting an emergency situation, one can only take time to check the obvious facts. The more one can tell the physician in the first phone call the better. For example, suppose the patient has been seriously burned. It would not be very helpful to the doctor to say, "Mr. B. has been burned." Some of the facts the doctor should be told include what caused the burn (heat—direct or indirect, chemical, electricity, steam, etc.); area of the body involved; extent of the burn; and, as far as is known, the depth of the burn. The

simplest way of judging and of expressing the depth of the burn is to use the degree classification; that is, first degree (reddening of the skin), second degree (blisters), and third degree (destruction of tissues below the skin).

A hypothetical case: "Mrs. C. has just been burned. Her dress caught on fire while she was using the gas stove. It was put out quickly and the burn does not appear to be very serious. However, there is redness over most of the left arm and side of the body. A few small blisters have appeared." These facts give the physician a fairly clear picture of what happened and what should be done for the patient.

Another case: "Mr. D. is having a severe nosebleed. He has had several nosebleeds off and on for some time, but this one is much more severe than usual. The measures we used previously (these could be told to the doctor) have not been effective." This report gives the physician an indication of what should be done as well as what has already been tried.

2. When giving a routine report, only symptoms or facts that differ from those given in previous reports need to be mentioned. To illustrate: Mrs. M., an elderly patient, has a mild form of diabetes mellitus. Her condition has been controlled for some time with anti-hyperglycemic agents. However, a check of the urine showed it to be 3+ when previously it had been negative or 1+ at the most. The physician should be informed of the change. But the nurse might check other things before phoning the doctor. Is the patient eating all of her diet? Does she appear drowsy or stuporous? Has she any gastrointestinal disturbances such as nausea, vomiting, loss of appetite, diarrhea, constipation? What are the vital signs? Including such information in the report will save valuable time for both the attendant and the doctor.

Of course, there are times when only a word or two is needed; for example, "Mrs. R. is doing very well although she complains of insomnia. The night attendant says she sleeps more than she realizes but, even so, she is not getting the normal amount of sleep that we feel she should."

3. Possibly the most difficult type of reporting is that required when the physician knows very little about the patient's condition at the time of the report. The doctor may not have seen the patient in several weeks or even months. It is not very helpful to report that "Mr. D. is not feeling very well today," or that "Mrs. M. has just

been admitted; what orders do you wish carried out for her?" These statements tell the physician practically nothing. He must ask many questions that the attendant cannot answer without going to the patient several times. This is a waste of everyone's time.

MEANINGFUL REPORTING

What facts should the attendant learn before he reports to the doctor? The following list of facts to be noted and charted before calling the doctor may include some that will not be needed in every case, and may omit some that may sometimes be needed, but it will serve as a guide:

Vital Signs

Temperature, pulse rate, respiration rate, and blood pressure. In emergencies and certain other conditions, the temperature report may be omitted.

Subjective Symptoms

Subjective symptoms are those complained of by the patient; for example, headache, backache, pain, nausea, "indigestion," and so on.

If the patient is conscious and rational, note the subjective symptoms first. Do not suggest symptoms by asking the patient whether he has a headache or pain, but ask a question such as "How are you?" or "How are you feeling today?" If he indicates some difficulty you might ask, "What seems to be the trouble?" This should bring out subjective symptoms without your suggesting any.

Objective Symptoms

Objective symptoms are those that an attendant can observe; for example, color of the lips and skin; any swellings, rashes, bruises, enlargement of joints, fracture deformities; external bleeding; state of consciousness; etc.

Objective symptoms involve close scrutiny, but they need not be too time-consuming. The attendant who gets the habit of observing patients closely and in a systematic way can obtain a great deal of information in a very few minutes. Some of the important things to note and record when abnormalities are observed include:

1. An overall picture: Does the patient look ill? Is there any predominant sign such as, for example, always preferring to lie on one side? If the patient is ambulatory, does he seem stable on his feet? Does he stand upright?

2. Color of the face, lips, and whites of the eyes.

3. Pupils of the eyes: Are they dilated, contracted, or normal and equal in size? Is there a lack of tears or excessive tearing?

4. Condition of the patient's hair: Is it ample and lustrous, or thin, dry, and brittle? Is the patient bald (in spots, or as occurs in aging)?

5. Condition of the mouth: Do the gums appear normal? What about the teeth? Do the patient's dentures seem to fit properly?

6. Respirations: Note rate, depth, type (chest or abdominal breathing or both), regularity or irregularity of breathing, and whether it is noisy, wheezing, or labored. Note type of cough, if present, and of expectoration (what is coughed up). Does the patient breathe through his nose, mouth, or both? Does he need to sit up to breathe?

7. Pulse: Note not only the rate but whether the beat is regular. If irregular, is a beat missed at regular or irregular intervals? Does the beat feel full or thin? Any other seeming abnormality?

8. Skin: Note general condition. Is there any rash, bruise, or edema and if so, where and how much?

9. Breasts: In the female, note whether the breasts seem to be normal in size, symmetry, and general appearance.

10. Abdomen: Note whether the abdomen is distended and ask the patient whether he has had any nausea, vomiting, diarrhea, or constipation recently. Does he have hemorrhoids?

11. Kidney function: Is the urine normal in color and amount? Insufficient? Excessive? Does the patient have to urinate frequently, with urgency, or during the night? (Once during the night may be considered normal.)

12. Genitalia: Note any abnormal discharge.

13. Muscles, bones, and joints: Are there any indications of arthritis? If so, where and how many joints are involved, and how badly? Do the patient's joints appear to function

normally? Are the muscles flabby? (This is not unusual in the elderly person.) Is the patient able to handle himself, that is, can he walk without help? If not, how much help does he need? If he is not ambulatory can he use a wheel-chair or is he confined to bed?

In summary, note and report everything that appears to you to be abnormal.

In the following hypothetical case a nursing home attendant is speaking to the physician.

Mr. A. has been admitted. We understand you have not seen the patient in several weeks, but sent him here because of an accident which has left no one at his home to care for him for the time being. His nephew, Mr. B., brought him to the home and, from our observation and what Mr. B. could tell us, the situation seems to be this:

Mr. A. is known to have a cardiac condition and is mildly decompensated. He brought his medications with him. (Here the attendant names the drugs and reports the instructions for taking them.) Mr. A. is now very confused and disoriented. He does not appear to be acutely ill. Vital signs are: temperature, 97.8° F; pulse, 90 (somewhat irregular with an occasional missed beat, volume fair); respirations, 20 and somewhat labored. He breathes best in a sitting position. Blood pressure, 190/80. Color is quite good; no cyanosis. We asked Mr. B. about the patient's gastrointestinal and kidney functions, but he could give us little information; however, there is no apparent malfunctioning of either system. The patient's skin is in generally good condition, but there is some pitting edema of the ankles.

This report gives the physician a fairly clear picture of the patient's condition and he can readily order new medications or treatment, or changes in the present regimen. His orders for this patient might well include such diagnostic procedures as urinalysis, complete blood count, and electrocardiogram. He probably would also order a hypnotic, since new surroundings are not conducive to rest and relaxation. Telephoned orders should be recorded on the patient's chart, and the physician should be asked to initial them when he first visits the patient so as to make them authentic.

MEDICATIONS FOR GERIATRIC PATIENTS

The administration of medications to older patients presents many problems not met with in younger patients. Some of these problems are physical in nature, some are emotional, and some are due to the actions of the drugs themselves.

Intestinal absorption is usually less than completely adequate in the older person. This should be remembered when a drug that is given orally does not have the expected results; pills with a hard coating or hard tablets may pass through the gastrointestinal tract unchanged and appear in the stools. In most cases, the elderly patient tolerates stimulants better than he does depressants; therefore, it is common practice to reduce the standard dosage of depressants for him unless he has been taking the drug for some time and has built up a tolerance for it. Also, the side effects of drugs are often more pronounced in the older person and may also be atypical. Consequently, any adverse symptoms that appear to be drug-induced should be reported promptly to the physician.

Some patients find it difficult to swallow tablets or pills. Unless very large, capsules are often easier to swallow than pills, because of their shape. Sometimes, a tablet or pill can be given with a little food, such as bread, instead of water. Or the tablet can be crushed and put into an empty capsule. Of course, delayed-reaction preparations must be administered in the form and manner ordered.

Administration of medications by injection often presents problems in the older patient. The elderly usually have less muscle mass than younger persons and this makes it difficult to give an injection subcutaneously or intramuscularly. Also, the older patient tends to be either edematous, obese, or emaciated and, in each case, intramuscular or subcutaneous injections may result in ecchymosis (escape of blood into tissues from ruptured blood vessels) or sterile abscesses more often than in the younger individual whose tissues are normal. When the patient has a tendency toward dependent edema, the buttocks should not be used for injection of drugs, because absorption from those tissues may be slow and incomplete.

There are many different emotional factors associated with medications for the elderly. In most cases, an elderly patient has been taking certain drugs for a long time, whether prescribed by a physician or not. Self-medication is a national habit of huge proportions. Most people do not think of laxatives, vitamins, cough preparations, and analgesics such as aspirin, or mild sedatives as medicines.

They think of "medicines" as drugs ordered by the physician, "drugs" as substances used by addicts, and the drugs they take "on their own" as simple remedies that make life a little more comfortable. While most of the drugs that can be purchased over the counter are not addictive, many of them are habit-forming, and, as is well-known, any attempt to change habits in older people is emotionally upsetting to them. When an older person enters an institution and is denied drugs not ordered by the attending physician, a stress situation may develop. The patient cannot understand why he cannot have the same drugs he has been taking at home. Attendants often overlook the fact that a prescribed drug may actually be the same as one the patient had been taking at home, but it appears different to him because it is not the same form or color, since different drug manufacturers use different forms and colors for their brands of medications that are all the same basic substance. As far as the patient is concerned, he is getting a different drug, and this can be very disturbing to him. Also, the patient may have maintained a certain schedule at home that is not followed in the hospital. For example, he may have used eye drops for glaucoma four times a day—6:00 and 10:00 a.m. and 6:00 and 10:00 p.m., which spaces the doses evenly throughout the 24 hours. But in many institutions medications ordered for four times a day are given at 8:00 a.m., 12:00 noon, and 4:00 and 8:00 p.m., and this allows a time interval of 12 hours without the drug. The patient usually knows that preservation of his sight is dependent upon the drops, and this change in the routine can be very upsetting.

The administration of medications is an extremely important aspect of patient care, and anyone who gives medications should be well informed about both the patient and the drugs that are ordered for him. The nurse should find out what medications the patient has been taking at home, and carefully explain any changes the doctor orders. It may be necessary to repeat the explanation several times.

PRESCRIPTIONS

A prescription is a kind of letter of instructions sent by the physician to a pharmacist. A standard form and abbreviations are used to save space and time. In the past, prescriptions were much more complicated and detailed than they are now, since the pharmacist compounded most of the medications himself. Now this is done in the pharmaceutical company laboratories. The medications arrive at the pharmacy in the form and dosage usually ordered. This has made prescription writing much simpler. Formerly, many drugs or chemicals were listed on the prescription; today it is rare for more than one substance to be named on any one prescription. A sample prescription follows (see also Appendix A, Medical Terminology, for definitions of the abbreviations used).

Name and address   Date

Mrs. H. G. Brown   12/10/75
810 Maple Avenue
Carronville, Iowa

R_X Digoxin 0.125 mg. #100

Sig. 1 tab. q.d.

rep. 2 times
☐ non rep.
☐ Do not drive, drink alcoholic beverages, or
    operate machinery while on this medication

D. O. Dunbar, M. D.   State License No. 82273
Medical Center Building Suite 15
1894 Main Avenue   DEA No. AD2988371
Carronville, Iowa

EXTENDED CARE IN THE HOME

When an elderly patient is very ill, it is usually best to have him treated in a hospital. But often, when the acute phase of an illness is over, it is possible for him to be cared for in his home. If possible, the room chosen for a patient at home should be relatively quiet and easily heated, cooled, and ventilated. It should be next to or near a bathroom. Throw rugs should be removed; a slip-proof, easy-to-clean, wall-to-wall carpet is preferable. Heavy draperies should be replaced with washable curtains.

The bed should be high enough that the person caring for the patient does not strain his back, but low enough for the patient to get into and out of easily. If the patient can touch the floor with his toes when sitting on the edge of the bed, the height is about right. If possible, the bed should be placed so that it can be approached from either side. The patient should be able to see out of a window, but direct (electric) light in the eyes should be avoided. A bedside stand on each side is helpful; a bedside lamp is a must. A clock with a luminous dial and large figures should be provided, and television with remote control and a radio will help to pass the time.

There should be a comfortable chair with armrests near the bed and a footstool if the chair is high, so that the patient's feet do not hang loose. A small table near the patient's chair will allow him to keep various objects he needs within reach, including a bell so that he can call for help when he needs it. If he cannot go to the family dining room an overbed table will be needed. In an emergency, such a table can easily be improvised by placing a wide, smooth board over the bed with the ends resting on the backs of two chairs or on books or bricks piled on either side of the bed. An overbed table or board can be used for such other things as grooming, writing, and so on.

Let the patient groom himself if he can manage this. Supply him with the necessary equipment, allow him to do what he can, and help him as needed. If he is in bed all or most of the time, a daily sponge bath and clean linen will help keep his skin in good condition, but if he is up most of the day a tub bath or shower every other day might be better. The tub should be made as accident-proof as possible and someone should remain within call while the patient is bathing.

The diet instructions will be given by the physician, nurse, or dietician. In most cases, the patient is better off with five or six small meals than three large ones. Unless limited by medical order, fluids are given in generous amounts; not just water but fluid foods as well. Elimination can usually be regulated by the foods the patient eats. Ample fluids will aid in kidney output, and laxative foods will help keep bowel action satisfactory. The physician may order 24-hour intake and output records kept in order to determine whether output is satisfactory; be sure to include the fluid foods as well as water. Output will usually not equal intake, since some fluid is lost through perspiration.

The person in charge of the patient would do well to keep a chart, including at least the following:

1. Daily temperature, taken at approximately the same time each day, unless otherwise ordered by the doctor.
2. Other vital signs, including pulse rate and respiration rate. If blood pressure readings are important, the physician or nurse will teach the individual taking care of the patient to do this. A clock or watch with a second hand is required for taking pulse and respirations. Locate the pulse by feeling the wrist just below the thumb; place the patient's arm so that the palm of the hand is down; rest the arm on the bed or on the patient's chest so that you can feel the patient's respiratory movements; count the pulse for one minute and then the respirations for one minute. Record your findings on the chart.
3. Medications are given at the times indicated on the prescriptions, and any drug effects that are seen should be recorded. Did the patient sleep after taking his sleeping pill? Was his pain relieved by the analgesic ordered?
4. Any unusual occurrence, physical or emotional, and any improvement or regression should be noted on the chart.
5. When the patient is allowed out of bed part of the time, his reaction to this activity should be noted. Did he need help to walk? Did he become overly tired?
6. Urination and defecation should be recorded.

Special precautions must be taken to prevent bedsores, contractures (shortening of muscle or tendon), and muscle atrophy (wasting away of the muscle) when the patient is confined to bed. Any number of problems may arise in patients who must remain in bed over an extended period of time. Care by a public health nurse will be most helpful; if this is not possible, a nurse or physician may be asked for instructions.

The ill person in the home needs stimulating interests just as much if not more than persons who are up and around. Radio, television, newspapers, magazines, and books are helpful. Even more valuable are visits from friends and participation in hobbies and crafts that can be done in bed or while sitting in a chair. But, by all means, regardless of how time-consuming and important the patient's physical needs may be, do not forget his social, psychological, and emotional needs.

SECTION II

Diseases and Disorders of the Elderly

The same diseases and disorders that affect young individuals are also seen in the elderly. However, as one grows older one is more likely to develop illnesses that are degenerative in nature.

In many parts of the world better maternal and child health care has greatly reduced the hazards of childbirth for both mothers and babies, and the infectious diseases of childhood have practically disappeared. Since the discovery of the causes of such infectious diseases as measles, diphtheria, poliomyelitis, smallpox, cholera, bubonic plague, and yellow fever, most people no longer live in fear of epidemics of these diseases. The causes of diabetes mellitus and pernicious anemia are also known, and, although these diseases cannot be cured, they can be controlled so that the patient can live a relatively normal life. Health teams are currently concentrating on the major killers and cripplers of today—cardiovascular disease, cancer, respiratory disorders, and arthritis. If the first two could be prevented or cured, life expectancy would be extended by several years; if arthritis could be overcome, those added years would be much more enjoyable.

Section II of this book contains descriptions of the diseases and disorders that most frequently affect older people; it does not presume to be complete. The entries have been classified according to the body system affected, since this is the common medical practice. No specific therapies are included, because they will be determined by the attending physician and the particular circumstances of each case. Suggested treatments are general in nature and usually differentiated as medical or surgical. Not every available diagnostic procedure is given; but the more common tests and procedures that can be carried out in almost every health facility, and often in the patient's home, are included.

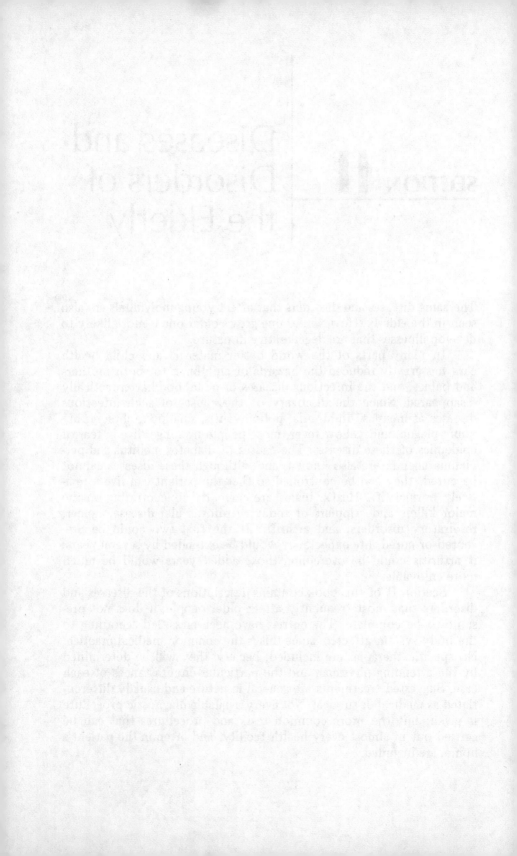

CHAPTER 1 | Diseases and Disorders of the Digestive System

THE GASTROINTESTINAL SYSTEM

Adenocarcinoma of the Rectum

Condition: A malignant tumor of the rectum.
Cause: Unknown. Polyps of the rectum appear to be a predisposing factor.
Symptoms and Signs: Changes in bowel habits; diarrhea and/or constipation, or these two symptoms may alternate; rectal pain; tenesmus; a feeling of fullness in the rectum; bloody stools; a malodorous discharge that contains blood, mucus, or pus, which may or may not appear with the stool. Rectal examination reveals an elevated, hard, irregular lesion.
Diagnostic Procedures Usually Ordered: Proctoscopy, biopsy, x-ray (barium enema).
Treatment: Usually, surgery. Otherwise, treatment is palliative and symptomatic.
Complications: Intestinal obstruction, hemorrhage, secondary fistulas into the bladder or through the skin. When diagnosed late, widespread metastases involving such structures as the sciatic nerve or the bladder.
Course: If surgery is ineffective, the course is progressive and fatal.

Anal Cryptitis

Condition: Inflammation of a crypt (pit, hair follicle, or glandular tubule) in the anal structures; may be multiple.
Cause: A bacterial infection.
Symptoms and Signs: Pain following defecation; pruritus (itching); possibly, blood-streaked stools or purulent discharge.
Treatment: *Conservative*—sitz baths, fecal softeners, mineral oil, analgesic-antiseptic suppositories. If conservative measures fail, dilation of the anal sphincter or surgery is called for.
Complication: Perianal abscess; anal fistula.

Anal Fissure

Condition: A longitudinal crack in the anal canal.
Causes: Constipation, diarrhea, bacterial infection, ulcerative colitis.
Treatment: As for anal cryptitis.

Anorectal Fistula

Condition: An abnormal opening between the rectum and the exterior.
Causes: Infection, cancer, intestinal tuberculosis, ulcerative colitis, trauma, extension of an abscess from an anal crypt.
Symptoms and Signs: Pain, inflammation of rectal and anal canals, rectal edema, purulent discharge.
Treatment: Chemotherapeutic agents may be tried, but surgery is necessary to correct the condition.
Complication: Ulceration; tendency to recurrence.

Carcinoma of the Colon
(including Adenocarcinoma)

Condition: A malignant tumor arising in the colon, usually in the sigmoid colon or in the ileocecal area.
Causes: Direct cause, unknown. Often associated with colonic polyps or ulcerative colitis.
Symptoms and Signs: A change in bowel habits, nausea, pallor, loss of weight. May be asymptomatic if the tumor is in the ileocecal area, but sometimes there is distention and/or pain in the lower abdomen. When the sigmoid is involved: abdominal pain, more pronounced on the left side; ribbon- or pencil-shaped stools; a palpable mass in the lower left quadrant; usually the lesion can be seen on proctoscopic examination.
Diagnostic Procedures Usually Ordered: Complete blood count, stool examination for occult blood, biopsy, x-ray (barium enema).
Treatment: Usually, surgery. When metastasis occurs, treatment is symptomatic and palliative.
Complications: Invasion of the pelvic organs by the tumor, metastasis to the liver or the regional lymph nodes, anemia, angina pectoris, cardiac insufficiency.
Course: The estimated five-year survival rate following removal of tumor is 70 percent if metastasis has not occurred; 30 percent if metastasis has occurred.

Carcinoma of the Esophagus

Condition: A malignant tumor of the esophagus; may occur in any part of the esophagus, but more than half occur in the lower third of the esophagus. Occurs more often in males than in females.

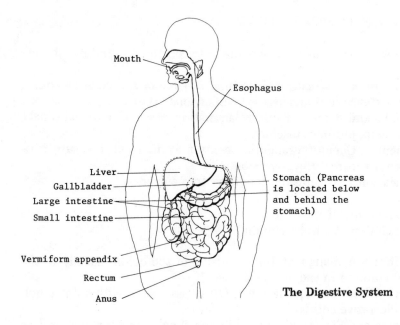

Mouth

Esophagus

Liver

Gallbladder

Large intestine

Small intestine

Stomach (Pancreas is located below and behind the stomach)

Vermiform appendix

Rectum

Anus

The Digestive System

Cause: Unknown. Precipitating factors: smoking, alcoholism, carcinoma of surrounding structures, stricture.

Symptoms and Signs: Substernal discomfort, back pain, cough and hoarseness, sense of fullness, progressive difficulty in swallowing, regurgitation.

Diagnostic Procedures Usually Ordered: Esophagoscopy, x-ray, biopsy.

Treatment: Surgical.

Complications: Metastasis to surrounding structures, liver, lungs.

Course: Estimated five-year survival rate is less than 10 percent.

Carcinoma of the Stomach

Condition: A malignant tumor of the stomach.

Cause: Unknown. Precipitating factors may include: chronic gastritis, peptic ulcer or polyps, familial tendency, pernicious anemia.

Symptoms and Signs: Often asymptomatic at first. Discomfort in the epigastric region, general weakness, loss of weight, anemia; sometimes jaundice.

Diagnostic Procedures Usually Ordered: Gastric fluid analysis, various blood tests, stool examination for occult blood, x-ray, biopsy; possibly, gastroscopy.

Treatment: Surgical.

Complications: Metastasis to surrounding structures, hemorrhage.

Course: Depends on effectiveness of treatment and type and degree of metastatic spread. When diagnosed and treated early, the estimated five-year survival rate is 70 percent.

Diarrhea (chronic)

Condition: Inflammation of the gastrointestinal tract characterized by frequent, copious evacuations.

Causes: Infection, acute enteritis, allergy, emotional strain, food and other poisonings, nontropical sprue. Accompanies cystic fibrosis in children.

Symptoms and Signs: Frequent, watery stools that contain large amounts of fat and bits of undigested food, may alternate with constipation; sense of fullness, distention, and/or pain in the abdomen; nausea after eating; dehydration and weight loss if untreated.

Diagnostic Procedure Usually Ordered: X-ray (barium enema).

Treatment: Removal of the cause, if possible; dietary regulation; otherwise, treatment is symptomatic.

Diverticulosis and Diverticulitis

Condition: *Diverticulosis*—the presence of multiple diverticula (outpouchings), particularly in the intestinal canal. Occurs most often in the sigmoid colon, but may also occur in the ileocecal area; rarely in the small bowel.

Diverticulitis—inflammation of one or more diverticula.

Cause: *Diverticulosis*—unknown; may be the result of intestinal infection that has weakened the intestinal muscle wall.

Diverticulitis—a bacterial infection that occurs when the opening of a diverticulum into the bowel is obstructed by edema, a fecalith, or other substance.

Symptoms and Signs: *Diverticulosis*—sometimes none. Low abdominal pain, usually in the left or right lower quadrant, or both, is common, as are periods of constipation alternating with diarrhea; sometimes, intolerance for foods high in roughage or gas-producing foods.

Diverticulitis—pain and tenderness in the area involved, sometimes accompanied by cramping, nausea, vomiting, and low fever.

Diagnostic Procedure Usually Ordered: X-ray (barium enema).
Treatment: *Diverticulosis*—usually none is required. Diarrhea and constipation are treated as usual.
    Diverticulitis—anti-infective drugs. If the condition is severe and there is danger of rupture, surgical resection of the affected portion of the bowel is indicated.
Complications: Diverticulitis, which is itself a complication of diverticulosis, may result in perforation of the intestinal wall and peritonitis, abscess formation, fistulation, hemorrhage, and intestinal obstruction.
Course: Diverticulosis has a chronic course, but it is not life-threatening. Diverticulitis has an acute course requiring medical or surgical treatment, to which it usually responds.

Dysentery (bacillary)

Condition: Infection of the intestinal tract, especially the large bowel.
Cause: An organism of the *Shigella* genus.
Symptoms and Signs: Abdominal pain and spasm in the lower portion of the intestinal tract, fever, diarrhea with the passage of mucus and blood, anorexia, weight loss, dehydration.
Diagnostic Procedures Usually Ordered: White blood cell count, stool culture, sigmoidoscopy.
Treatment: The appropriate antibiotic drug, isolation of the patient.
Complication: Ulceration of the large bowel.
Course: Onset is abrupt. The diarrhea is usually self-limited.

Dysphagia Sideropenia

Other Name: Plummer-Vinson syndrome.
Condition: Difficulty in swallowing due to atrophy in the mouth, pharynx, and upper end of the esophagus.
Cause: Exact cause unknown. Precipitating factors: vitamin and iron deficiencies appear in most cases.
Symptoms and Signs: The condition is accompanied by anemia, glossitis, and stomatitis.
Treatment: Iron therapy and supplemental vitamins as indicated.

Esophageal Diverticulum

Other Name: Zenker's diverticulum.
Condition: An outpouching of the esophagus; may be single or multiple.
Cause: Usually unknown.
Symptoms and Signs: Dysphagia, regurgitation of food and fluids.
Diagnostic Procedures Usually Ordered: X-ray, esophagoscopy.
Treatment: Mechanical dilatation if the condition is due to a stricture; otherwise, surgical.
Complications: Aspiration pneumonia, malnutrition.
Course: Depends on efficacy of treatment.

Esophagitis (chronic, peptic)

Condition: Chronic inflammation of the esophagus, characterized by regurgitation of gastric contents.
Causes: Congenital anomaly, esophageal hiatal hernia, frequent vomiting, prolonged use of nasogastric tubes; possibly, a complication following gastric surgery.
Symptoms and Signs: Difficulty in swallowing; heartburn; regurgitation of gastric chyme, often with hemorrhage.
Treatment: Remove the cause, if possible; otherwise, symptomatic.

Gastrointestinal Hemorrhage

Condition: Not a disease entity but a symptom that consists of bleeding in some portion of the gastrointestinal tract.
Causes: Peptic ulcer, gastritis, gastric or intestinal polyps, rupture of esophageal varices, predisposition to hemorrhage, hiatal hernia, rupture of Meckel's diverticulum, carcinoma in any part of the tract, tuberculosis of the colon, hookworm, uremia, infection of the intestinal tract.
Symptoms and Signs: Hematemesis if the bleeding is in the esophagus or stomach, tarry stools (melena) if the bleeding is in the upper intestinal tract or stomach (if blood is not vomited), occult blood in the stools if bleeding is in the lower intestine. In cases of mild bleeding, blood in stools may be detected only by laboratory methods. In severe hemorrhage: coldness; moist, clammy skin; restlessness; pallor

or cyanosis (especially of the fingers); hypotension; rapid, thready pulse; reduced urine output.

Treatment: Removal of the cause. Transfusion if the hemorrhage is severe.

Complication: Prolonged bleeding, even in small amounts, may result in anemia.

Course: Depends entirely on the cause and severity of the hemorrhage, and effectiveness of the treatment.

Glossitis

Condition: Inflammation of the tongue; several varieties are recognized.

Causes: Many: Infection, chemical or thermal burns, excessive smoking or chewing of tobacco, dental disorders (including misfitting dentures).

Symptoms and Signs: In acute glossitis there may be pain, fever, salivation, and swelling of the tongue. In the form known as Moeller's glossitis, red patches appear on the sides and tip of the tongue, and there may be burning or pain of the tongue, sensitivity to spicy foods, and disturbance of the sense of taste. In the form known as smokers' patch, thin, crinkly, pearly lesions appear which later become thick and creamy-white and desquamate, leaving a beefy red base.

Treatment: Removal of the cause, correction of dental mechanism if needed, anti-infectives for local and/or systemic infections.

Course: Remissions and relapses are apt to occur.

Hemorrhoids

Condition: A varicose vein (or veins) in the mucous membrane inside the rectum (internal hemorrhoids) or at the very lower end of the rectum and at the anus (external hemorrhoids).

Causes: Infections, constipation, straining at stool, portal obstruction, ulcerative colitis, heavy lifting, pregnancy, increased intra-abdominal pressure, tumor. In some cases, unknown.

Symptoms and Signs: Rectal pain, especially on defecation; pruritus.

Internal hemorrhoids—bleeding and protrusion of the lesions through the anal opening with defecation, abdominal straining, or heavy lifting; possibly, prolapse of the hemorrhoids.

External hemorrhoids—multiple, rounded, purplish, thrombosed

lesions; edema of the anal tissues; ulceration; sloughing; possibly, bleeding and/or gangrene.
Diagnostic Procedure Usually Ordered: Proctoscopy.
Treatment: Astringent and analgesic suppositories; sometimes, surgery. Small hemorrhoids may not require treatment.
Complications: Strangulation   of   the   hemorrhoid,   malignant changes, anemia due to chronic blood loss.
Course: Depends on the size of the hemorrhoids and the effectiveness of the treatment. Recurrences are common.

Hiatal Hernia

Other Names: Diaphragmatic hernia, paraesophageal hernia, sliding hernia.
Condition: A portion of the abdominal contents (usually the stomach) protrudes upward through the esophageal hiatus in the diaphragm.
Causes: Usually a congenital anomaly. May result from trauma.
Symptoms and Signs: Many, but they do not always indicate the trouble. Dyspnea, hiccups, vomiting, dysphagia, palpitation, epigastric pain that is usually worse after eating or when lying down. Sometimes, cyanosis, peristaltic sounds in the chest, retrosternal pain that may be interpreted by the patient as cardiac in origin.
Diagnostic Procedure Usually Ordered: X-ray. It is important to differentiate between a hiatal hernia and a heart attack.
Treatment: Surgery, if the patient's condition warrants it. Several small meals a day instead of three large ones; avoidance of the recumbent position for 2 hours after eating; abstinence from food for 2 hours before retiring; if necessary, elevation of the head of the bed on 6-inch blocks to prevent regurgitation of food at night; antacids for relief of pain.
Complications: Peptic esophagitis, cardiac or respiratory disturbances due to pressure in the chest cavity, pneumonitis from regurgitation of food.
Course: Chronic. Final outcome depends on effectiveness of treatment.

Intestinal Obstruction and Ileus

Condition: *Intestinal obstruction* is a blockage (partial or complete) that interferes with the passage of feces along the intestinal tract. *Ileus* is a condition characterized by lack of intestinal motility that prevents the feces from moving normally along the intestinal tract.

Causes: *Obstruction*—many and varied. In young children the cause may be directly related to age. In adults common causes include hernia, postoperative adhesions, gallstones or enteroliths, worms, compression of the intestinal wall by tumor, foreign bodies, intussusception, kinking of the bowel.

Ileus—lack of effective peristalsis may be due to disturbances of the autonomic nervous system; often associated with peritonitis.

Symptoms and Signs: Vary with the degree, location, and duration of the obstruction. Intermittent abdominal pain (especially in the area around the umbilicus); fever; abdominal distention (less noticeable in jejunal than in other types of ileus), which may be localized in colonic obstruction. Rumbling noises that increase with the pain are heard in mechanical obstruction, but not in ileus. If strangulation occurs: tenderness and rigidity of the abdominal wall, dehydration, and shock may indicate developing peritonitis.

Diagnostic Procedures Usually Ordered: X-ray, blood chemistry.

Treatment: For mechanical obstruction or strangulation, surgery. For ileus, treatment of the underlying cause; use of a nasogastric tube may be necessary.

Complications: Perforation and peritonitis, electrolyte imbalance from nausea and vomiting.

Course: Depends chiefly on the correction of the underlying cause.

Leukoplakia

Other Names: Smokers' patches, psoriasis of the mouth.

Condition: The occurrence of characteristic patches on the mucous membranes of the mouth and tongue.

Cause: May not be known. Known causes include trauma; irritation from dental restorations or from chemicals, including some drugs, tobacco, and thermal agents.

Symptoms and Signs: Local pain; typical grayish-white, leathery lesions with erythematous edges on the membranes of the cheeks and floor of the mouth and on the tongue. Later the lesions become ulcerated and fissured.

Diagnostic Procedure Usually Ordered: Biopsy.

Treatment: Elimination of the cause, if known, is all that may be needed. Excision of the lesions if single or few in number.

Complications: Malignancy is the most common and serious complication.

Course: Leukoplakia is considered precancerous.

Mesenteric Vascular Insufficiency Syndrome

Other Name: Mesenteric thrombosis.
Condition: A thrombus within a mesenteric blood vessel.
Causes: A thrombus may develop at the site of a lesion in the mesentery or in another part of the body, or develop as a complication of diverticulosis, appendicitis, trauma, or inflammatory pelvic disease.
Symptoms and Signs: *Acute form*—generalized, continuous abdominal pain; fever; constipation; shock.
   Chronic form—pain in the umbilical area, especially after eating, which may or may not be continuous; nausea and vomiting; diarrhea; possibly, constipation; abdominal distention and tenderness; loss of weight.
Diagnostic Procedures Usually Ordered: White blood cell count, differential count, examination of stool for occult blood, analysis of peritoneal fluid, x-ray.
Treatment: Usually surgical.
Complications: Intestinal perforation and/or peritonitis.
Course: Onset is acute. Course depends on condition of the patient and effectiveness of treatment.

Peptic Ulcer Syndrome

Condition: Erosion and ulceration of an area of the mucosa of the esophagus, stomach, or duodenum.
Causes: Many and varied. Underlying cause probably the inability of the gastrointestinal mucosa to withstand the proteolytic action of the acid in the gastric juice. Possible contributing factors include vascular states related to stasis and congestion; emotional stresses causing hyperacidity and hypermotility; administration of or excessive production of adrenocorticosteroids; chemical burns; diseases or surgery of the brain.
Symptoms and Signs: Pain; may be dull to sharp, according to the location and size of the ulcer; is felt in the substernal or subxiphoid area in esophageal ulcer, in the upper quadrant or left of the midline in gastric ulcer, and to the right of the midline between the umbilicus and the xiphoid or above the umbilicus in duodenal ulcer; is usually relieved by eating, especially alkaline or fatty foods; is intensified by acidic and spicy foods, alcohol, or nicotine. Other symptoms: tenderness, nausea, vomiting; possibly, a palpable mass over the area of the ulcer.
Diagnostic Procedures Usually Ordered: Gastric secretion tests and

analysis, gastroscopy, stool examination for occult blood, x-rays (gastric series).

Treatment: Conservative at first; if no improvement follows treatment, or if bleeding occurs, surgery may be indicated. If perforation occurs, surgery is mandatory.

Complications: Perforation, hemorrhage, anemia.

Course: Usually chronic, with long-term medical treatment. The syndrome is considered malignant or precancerous until proved otherwise.

Perianal Abscess

Condition: An abscess in the tissue surrounding the anus.

Causes: Infection of an anal gland, a thrombosed hemorrhoid, cancer, trauma.

Symptoms and Signs: Feeling of discomfort and weight in the rectum, rectal pain that increases on defecation, discomfort when walking or sitting; malaise; usually, a palpable lump at the margin of the anus.

Diagnostic Procedures Usually Ordered: White blood cell count, proctoscopy.

Treatment: Surgical incision and drainage.

Complication: See anal fissure.

Course: Surgery is usually curative.

Prolapse of the Rectum

Condition: The mucous membrane of the rectum protrudes through the anus in varying degrees; condition described as incomplete or partial, complete, or concealed.

Causes: Disease or injury to the pelvic structures that support the rectum, excessive straining.

Symptoms and Signs: The mucous membrane lining of the intestine protrudes through the anus, especially during defecation.

Treatment: If prolapse occurs only when defecating, manual reinsertion may be all that is necessary. For more severe prolapse, surgical repair of the weakened musculature is required.

Complications and Course: Usually satisfactory adjustment can be made by training patient in manual replacement; if this is not possible, surgical removal or cauterization may be required.

Sphincter Ani (incontinence)

Condition: Inability to control evacuation of rectal contents. More common in older persons who are bedridden than in those who are ambulatory.
Causes: Paralysis resulting from disease or injury to the nervous system; injury to the sphincter muscles by accident or surgery; severe systemic conditions such as typhoid fever, diabetes mellitus, shock, or coma; old age.
Symptoms and Signs: Involuntary passage of feces; may be transient or permanent, depending on the causative agent.
Treatment: If it is known and is remediable, the underlying condition should be treated; use of a fecal softener if the stools are hard; use of a commode rather than a bedpan.
Complications and Course: When condition is due to serious systemic disease, the incontinence is apt to be transient; when it is due to anorectal resection, it is apt to be permanent.

Sprue (nontropical)

Other Names: Adult celiac disease, adult idiopathic steatorrhea.
Condition: A nutritional disturbance characterized by reduction in the absorption of fats and fat-soluble vitamins through the intestinal mucosa; other nutritional substances may also be absorbed in less than normal amounts.
Causes: The interference of the protein fraction of gluten (wheat flour) with the proper absorption of certain food products.
Symptoms and Signs: Abdominal distention that disappears during sleep, glossitis, tympanitis, intermittent diarrhea, foul-smelling stools, bleeding, extreme lassitude, fatigue, fractures, tetany.
Diagnostic Procedures Usually Ordered: Stool examination; blood cholesterol level; examination of urine for urobilinogen; analysis of gastric contents.
Treatment: A gluten-free diet.
Complications: Dehydration; dermatitis; edema of the legs.
Course: Administration of folic acid, vitamin B_{12}, and antibiotics may result in remissions.

Stomatitis

Condition: Inflammation of the mucous membranes lining the mouth; most often occurs in debilitated persons.

Cause: Unknown. Precipitating factors thought to be infections, local erosion or abrasion, chemicals, dental caries, or accumulation of tartar.

Symptoms and Signs: Painful yellowish, depressed, spherical lesions with red margins that begin at the margin of the gum and spread to the cheek and lower side of the tongue; enlargement of nearby lymph glands; salivation; coated tongue; putrid breath odor.

Treatment: Adequate diet with vitamin supplements; meticulous oral hygiene, with dental restoration and repair if needed; appropriate antibiotic therapy.

Complication: Ulceration that may extend to the alveolar process and result in necrosis of the bone.

Course: Antibiotic therapy may be helpful.

THE GALLBLADDER

Cholecystitis (chronic)

Condition: Chronic inflammation of the gallbladder.

Causes: Usually obscure; could be a primary infection, perpetuation of an attack of acute cholecystitis, or the result of cholelithiasis.

Symptoms and Signs: Often vague and ill defined. Usually, intolerance to fatty foods; belching; discomfort after eating; regurgitation; tenderness in the upper right abdominal quadrant; nausea; vomiting; colic; pain.

Diagnostic Procedure Usually Ordered: X-ray (gastrointestinal series) after oral or intravenous administration of a dye to show gallstones.

Treatment: Depends on age and physical condition of the patient, and whether he is jaundiced or has gallstones. Patients over 80 years of age who are not jaundiced are usually best left alone. Surgery is indicated for the younger patient if gallstones are present. For all patients, the diet should be low in fats.

Complications: Choleliths may cause obstruction of the common bile duct or damage the bile duct or the gallbladder. Another complication may be cirrhosis of the liver.

Course: If mild, the condition may persist for years, since the inflammation rarely subsides. If stones are present the condition usually worsens progressively.

Cholelithiasis

Other Names: Gallstones, gallbladder calculi.
Causes: Some dysfunction in the biliary system, possibly resulting from a disturbance of metabolism, infection, stasis, or obstruction. Other possibilities include: mechanical stasis of the organs of the biliary system, malignancy in the biliary tract, any long-standing disease of the gallbladder.
Symptoms and Signs: Usually, intermittent pain under the right shoulder blade or in the epigastric region; tenderness in the upper right quadrant of the abdomen; jaundice, in cases of obstruction; intolerance to fatty foods; nausea; vomiting; heartburn; regurgitation; flatulence or a sensation of fullness in the upper abdomen. Sometimes there are no symptoms or signs.
Diagnostic Procedures Usually Ordered: X-ray (gastrointestinal series) following oral or intravenous administration of dye to show possible gallstones; aspiration of duodenal fluid for analysis.
Treatment: See chronic cholecystitis.
Complications: If untreated, complications include cholecystitis, choledocholithiasis, hepatic disease, biliary cirrhosis, fistula, or ileus.
Course: If treated surgically, the outlook is usually good.

THE PANCREAS

Pancreatitis (acute, including acute hemorrhagic and acute interstitial forms)

Condition: Acute inflammation of the pancreas.
Causes: *Both forms*—often caused directly by excessive intake of alcohol or by dietary excess.

Acute hemorrhagic form—the escape of destructive enzymes from the small tubules of the pancreas into the substance of the gland; possibly, the rupture of canaliculi or shock (as occurs in myocardial infarction).

Acute interstitial form—may be unknown. Possible causes: infection, ingestion of toxic substances. Often associated with chronic cholecystitis.
Symptoms and Signs: *Acute hemorrhagic form*—sudden severe pain in the upper abdomen, radiating to the back and possibly to the

chest; nausea and vomiting; abdominal distention; jaundice; constipation resulting from decreased peristalsis.

Acute interstitial form—same as for the acute hemorrhagic form, plus prostration, fever, tachycardia, and transient jaundice.

Diagnostic Procedures Usually Ordered: White blood cell count, differential count, blood chemistry, upper gastrointestinal or abdominal x-ray.

Treatment: Much the same for both forms.

Emergency treatment—treatment for shock if it is present or appears to be developing, a strong analgesic for pain, atropine sulfate to control spasm, withholding fluid and food by mouth and giving what is needed intravenously.

Later treatment—usually, medical (conservative) treatment is preferred; that is, continuation of emergency treatment plus gastric suction for 48 to 72 hours, and symptomatic treatment as required.

Surgical treatment—used only when medical treatment fails or when it appears necessary to correct obstruction of a duct by stones, pancreatic abscess, or a complicating perforated peptic ulcer, or some similar disorder.

Complications: For both forms: shock, pancreatic abscess, necrotizing pancreatitis, pseudocyst formation, diabetes mellitus, insufficient secretion of pancreatic secretion, chronic pancreatitis.

Course: Recurrences are common, with about 10 percent of cases developing chronic pancreatitis. Mortality rate is over 10 percent with conservative treatment, higher if surgery is required.

Pancreatitis (chronic)

Condition: The recurrence of symptoms of acute pancreatitis at irregular intervals; begins usually in the third or fourth decade but may extend into the later years. More common in men than in women.

Causes: Varied; repeated attacks of acute pancreatitis, prolonged use of alcohol, pancreatic calculi.

Symptoms and Signs: Severe upper abdominal and back pain; vomiting; low grade fever; frequent, frothy, foul-smelling stools with high fat content; possibly, jaundice from obstruction of duct by calculi.

Diagnostic Procedures Usually Ordered: Serum amylase and lipase determinations, stool examination for fat and trypsin content, x-ray and arteriography of pancreas.

Treatment: Removal of predisposing cause if possible; bland, low fat diet; pancreatic enzymes with antacids or with food; narcotics used sparingly; alcohol is contraindicated; bile salts to aid digestion of fat. Surgery may be indicated to restructure the duct if the disease is of long standing and there has been extensive fibrosis of the pancreatic tissues.

CHAPTER 2

Diseases and Disorders of the Respiratory System

Bronchial Asthma

Condition: An allergic condition characterized by paroxysmal dyspnea, with wheezing and a sense of constriction in the chest.

Causes: *Extrinsic factors*: specific allergenic substances or nonspecific irritants such as pollens, animal dander, feathers, fungal spores, house dust, insecticides, glue, or lint; occasionally, ingestion of certain foods or drugs.

Intrinsic factors: usually, another infection of the respiratory tract (to which bronchial asthma is secondary); disturbances of the autonomic nervous system; possibly, emotional disturbances that aggravate the causative agent and increase the severity of the disease.

Symptoms and Signs: Paroxysmal attacks of wheezing, dyspnea, orthopnea, and sense of suffocation or pressure in the chest, most apt to occur at night, often precipitated by emotional experiences or exertion; early, a nonproductive cough; later, productive cough with expectoration of thick, stringy, mucoid sputum; debilitation and fatigue.

Diagnostic Procedures Usually Ordered: White blood cell count, differential count, sputum examination, chest x-ray.

Treatment:

(1)   Care during the attack: administration of sympathomimetic drugs such as epinephrine (Adrenalin), a xanthine preparation such as aminophylline, and a sedative; cough medicines as indicated; maintenance of the patient's general health with ample fluid intake and light, nourishing diet.

(2)   Finding the causative agent and removing it.

(3)   Preventing attacks by carrying out (2) and by administering drugs such as those used in treating acute attacks, but in smaller dosages.

Status asthmaticus, a severe form of asthma that does not respond to usual therapy, constitutes an emergency that requires hospitalization and energetic treatment.

Complications: Bronchitis, pneumonia, emphysema, pulmonary heart disease.

Course: Chronic, with remissions and exacerbations of varying lengths. When caused by extrinsic factors, the condition begins in childhood or early adulthood; when caused by intrinsic factors, it is most commonly seen first in middle or old age.

Bronchiectasis

Condition: Diffuse local inflammation with dilatation of the bronchioles; only one small area may be affected, or one lobe, or scattered areas over a large part of the lung.

Causes: Infections such as bronchopneumonia or tuberculosis; mucoviscidosis; aspiration of a foreign body; congenital anomaly; bronchial obstruction. May be the result of, or accompany, bronchial carcinoma or adenoma, or be a complication of agammaglobulinemia.

Symptoms and Signs: Vary with the extent and location of the affected area. When only small areas are involved, particularly if they are in the upper lobes, the patient may be asymptomatic (show no symptoms). When bases of the lungs are involved, usual symptoms include cough with abundant yellowish, chunky, foul sputum; hemoptysis; syncope; vomiting during coughing episodes; dyspnea; thoracic pain; clubbing of fingers and toes; limited chest expansion. Auscultatory signs: decrease in breath sounds; moist rales, most marked before expectoration. Chest is dull to percussion.

Diagnostic Procedures Usually Ordered: Chest x-ray, sputum examination; possibly, bronchoscopy.

Treatment: Measures to improve patient's general health, postural drainage to aid in removal of sputum (see Appendix H, Postural Drainage Exercises), surgical incision of lesions that are localized if patient's condition warrants (surgery not usually advised for the elderly). Use of a vaporizer may contribute to patient's comfort.

Medical treatment—Appropriate anti-infective drugs following report of sputum culture, antianemic drugs when indicated, expectorants, bronchodilators.

Complications: Pleurisy, pulmonary abscess, emphysema, anemia, sinusitis.

Course: Chronic. Relapses are common and are treated as required.

Bronchitis (acute and chronic) and Tracheitis

Condition: Inflammation of the trachea and bronchial tubes; may be isolated or part of a wider respiratory disease involving either the upper or lower respiratory tract, or both.

Causes: *Acute bronchitis*—usually, a viral or bacterial infection; may also be due to allergy, chemical or physical irritation, or presence of a foreign body.

Chronic bronchitis—same as for acute bronchitis; in addition, may be caused or intensified by smog, smoking, a cold damp climate, or repeated attacks of sinusitis, pneumonia, asthma, or bronchiectasis.

Tracheitis—infection, ingestion of a poison, presence of a foreign body.

Symptoms and Signs: *Acute bronchitis*—chills, fever, malaise, headache, generalized aches, cough, expectoration; sometimes, dyspnea; possibly, bilateral coarse moist rales.

Chronic bronchitis—cough, sometimes paroxysmal, with increasing expectoration of tenacious white or yellowish sputum; dyspnea may indicate oncoming or existing emphysema.

Tracheitis—dyspnea, fever, myalgia, malaise, rasping cough; feeling of rawness in the trachea and substernal oppression, which is aggravated by breathing cold air.

Diagnostic Procedures Usually Ordered: White blood cell count, differential count, sedimentation rate, chest x-ray; possibly, sputum examination.

Treatment: *Acute bronchitis*—bed rest, analgesics, steam inhalations, antitussives, appropriate antibiotics if causative agent is known.

Chronic bronchitis—underlying cause is treated as may be required; maintenance of the patient's general health; antitussives for nonproductive or severe cough; bronchodilators or antibiotics when indicated.

Tracheitis—when caused by presence of a foreign body, removal of foreign body is imperative; otherwise, treatment is same as for acute bronchitis.

Complications: *Acute bronchitis*—sinusitis, otitis media, bronchopneumonia.

Chronic bronchitis—purulent bronchitis, emphysema, bronchiectasis.

Tracheitis—tracheal edema, with partial or complete closure of the trachea; bronchitis.

Course: *Acute bronchitis*—usually self-limiting, lasting from a few days to several weeks, depending on severity of the disease and condition of the patient.

Chronic bronchitis—depends on the underlying cause, whether complications are present, and effectiveness of the treatment.

Tracheitis—same as for acute bronchitis.

Carcinoma of the Lungs (bronchiogenic carcinoma, adenocarcinoma of the lungs)

Condition: A malignant tumor in lung tissue.

Causes: There may be no apparent cause. Air pollution and inhalation of tobacco smoke are believed to be possible precipitating factors, but adenocarcinoma is apparently not due to these causes.

Symptoms and Signs: Early, there is a dry, irritating cough, which becomes productive with mucoid sputum, sometimes blood-tinged; chest pain; hemoptysis; loss of weight; nocturnal sweats; dysphonia; fever. Auscultatory signs include change in breath sounds, wheezing.

Diagnostic Procedures Usually Ordered: Chest x-ray, sputum examination; possibly, biopsy.

Treatment: Surgical incision if there are no known metastatic tumors and the patient's condition warrants it. Radiation may slow the progress of the disease; x-ray, radioactive cobalt, or the linear accelerator may be used. Aspiration to relieve effusions. Anticancer chemotherapeutic agents may be tried. Other treatment is supportive and palliative.

Complications: Many, including emphysema, pericarditis, superior vena cava syndrome, pulmonary abscess.

Course: Onset is insidious. Survival rate without surgery is relatively low; only 3 to 8 percent live 5 years or longer. Survival is shorter in adenocarcinoma. Metastasis to the brain, liver, and adrenal glands is common.

Coccidioidomycosis

Common Names: Valley fever, desert fever, San Joaquin fever.

Condition: Lesions similar to those of tuberculosis form in the lung tissue.

Cause: A fungus.

Symptoms and Signs: Nonproductive cough, anorexia, weight loss, night sweats, chest pain.

Diagnostic Procedures Usually Ordered: Skin test, sputum test, complement fixation test.

Treatment: Supportive and palliative; administration of antifungal drugs.

Complications and Course: Rarely, dissemination; fungating lesions; destructive lymphadenopathy.

Deviated Septum

Condition: The septum of the nose is bent to one side, partially or entirely blocking one nostril; is usually corrected in earlier life.
Treatment: Surgical, but only if the condition seriously affects the patient's breathing.

Emphysema

Condition: Dilatation of the air sacs of the lungs and loss of elasticity of lung tissue, increased resistance to the flow of air, regional difference in blood, and alteration of the response to stimulation by carbon dioxide.
Causes: Many, singly or in combination, or cause may be unknown. Predisposing factors: heredity; bronchial infections; chronic pulmonary disease such as bronchitis, pulmonary fibrosis, pneumoconiosis, pulmonary vascular disease, tuberculosis, or bronchoalveolitis; allergy; asthma; inhalation of toxic material such as atmospheric pollution or tobacco smoke; any interference with normal ventilation that causes obstruction.
Symptoms and Signs: (The patient may show no symptoms, especially in the early stage.) Barrel-shaped chest with limited respiratory movement, cough, dyspnea, cyanosis, anorexia, loss of weight. Rales may be heard on auscultation.
Diagnostic Procedures Usually Ordered: Breathing tests for vital capacity, blood tests for oxygen and carbon dioxide content, chest x-ray and/or fluoroscopy.
Treatment: The patient should be taught breathing exercises and encouraged to breathe deeply and to expectorate in order to remove as much sputum as possible (see Appendix G, Breathing Exercises for Home Use); tracheostomy may be required; oxygen, intermittently and in low concentrations. Other symptoms are treated as they occur.
    Medical treatment—anti-infective drugs for secondary infections, tranquilizers, sedatives, and hypnotics as needed.
Complications: Aggravation of the pulmonary pathology, right heart failure, spontaneous pneumothorax, peptic ulcer.
Course: Chronic. Electrolyte imbalance may occur, resulting in too much carbon dioxide in the arterial blood and not enough oxygen to meet the body's metabolic needs.

Laryngitis

Condition: Inflammation of the larynx; may be acute or chronic.
Causes: Viral or bacterial infection involving the upper respiratory
tract, improper or excessive use of the voice, inhalation of irritating
industrial fumes or gases, allergy, excessive use of alcohol or tobacco,
postnasal drip.
Symptoms and Signs: Raw, tickling, or burning sensation in the
throat; hoarseness; malaise; fever; possibly, loss of voice and dyspnea.
Treatment: See tonsillitis.

Massive Collapse of the Lung

Condition: Collapse of the air sacs and airlessness of the lung resulting from the obstruction of one of the bronchi by a mucus plug
or other object.
Causes: Carcinoma, chronic bronchitis, inhalation of a foreign
body; possibly, a complication of surgery.
Symptoms and Signs: Similar to those of spontaneous pneumothorax. Additionally, mediastinal structures are displaced toward the
affected side.
Treatment: Removal of the plug by bronchoscopy. Coughing and
deep breathing are encouraged and the patient is turned frequently
to prevent atelectasis. Other therapy is palliative and supportive.
Complications: Pneumonia, respiratory depression.
Course: Depends on whether the cause can be, and is, eliminated.

Nasal Polyp

Condition: A benign tumor of the nasal mucosa. May be single or
multiple.
Causes: Inflammation; allergic rhinitis.
Symptoms and Signs: Sneezing; nosebleed; postnasal drip; rhinor-
rhea; loss of sense of smell.
Diagnostic Procedures Usually Ordered: Microscopic examination
of nasal secretions for eosinophiles.
Treatment: Surgical, but usually only if the polyp causes repeated
nosebleeds or interferes with breathing.
Complications: Recurrence; sinusitis.
Course: When small there are no symptoms; may recur after surgi-
cal removal.

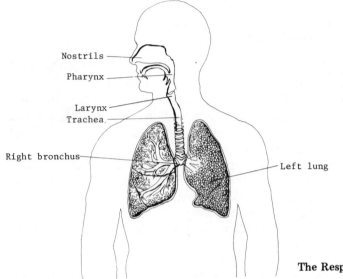

Nostrils

Pharynx

Larynx
Trachea

Right bronchus

Left lung

The Respiratory System

Pharyngitis (acute, chronic, sicca)

Common Name: Sore throat.

Condition: Inflammation of the pharynx, most often seen in the fall and winter.

Cause: Viral or bacterial infection. Sometimes associated with a more widespread upper respiratory infection.

Symptoms and Signs: *In all forms*—dryness, soreness, and redness of the throat; fever; malaise.

   Chronic—may be few symptoms other than cough with thick mucous exudate, throat pain, swelling.

   Sicca—very dry throat.

Treatment: *For all forms*—largely symptomatic (any underlying pathology should be treated): mild analgesics, throat irrigations, gargles, appropriate anti-infective drugs if the causative bacterium or virus has been identified.

Complication: Extension to the larynx, trachea, or bronchial tubes.

Course: Usually short except for the chronic form, but may persist until the underlying pathology is corrected or controlled.

The Pneumonias [Lobar, atypical (viral), and
aspiration pneumonia; bronchopneumonia
(lobular pneumonia), and pneumonitis]

Condition: Inflammation of the air sacs of the lungs; may be localized in one lobe or generalized throughout the lung tissue.
Causes: *Lobar pneumonia*—usually an infectious agent; pneumococcus is more commonly the cause in younger persons, staphylococcus is more commonly the cause in older persons; Friedlander's bacillus; Hemophilus influenzae.

Atypical (viral) pneumonia—an adenovirus called Eaton's agent.

Aspiration pneumonia—the aspiration of foreign material into
the lung (most common in debilitated patients who cannot clear
secretions from the throat and bronchi).

Bronchopneumonia—usually secondary to a viral or bacterial
infection; may also result from long confinement to bed.

Pneumonitis—a streptococcus.

Symptoms and Signs: First symptom in the elderly may be confusion; then malaise, dyspnea, persistent cough, pleuritic pain (rare in
atypical—viral—pneumonia); fever, 102 to 105°F, if untreated; cyanosis. Auscultatory signs include pleural friction rub, increased tactile and vocal fremitus, crepitant rales, bronchial breath sounds. Sputum is watery and turbid, later purulent and blood-tinged.

Atypical (viral) pneumonia—as above, plus bradycardia, inflammation of nasal and pharyngeal mucosa.

Aspiration pneumonia—regurgitation of stomach contents, nasal
secretions, fluids, bits of food, and medications.

Diagnostic Procedures Usually Ordered: White blood cell count,
differential count, sedimentation rate, sputum examination, chest
x-ray.

Treatment: Treatment includes bed rest, keeping the patient warm;
providing fluid intake of 2 to 3 liters each 24 hours, orally if possible, otherwise subcutaneously, rectally, or intravenously (intake
and output records are important); encouraging the patient to
breathe deeply, cough, and expectorate, and to change his position
frequently (Fowler's position is most comfortable); using foam rubber wedges under patient's heels to prevent decubitus ulcers; keeping
the legs extended, watching for signs of thromboembolism, and applying antiembolic stockings when indicated; encouraging ambula-
tion when temperature is normal; assisting the patient with active
and passive exercises; providing a light and nourishing diet. It is best

not to treat the elderly patient with pneumonia in a hospital because of the danger of acquiring a hospital-borne staphylococcal infection.

In aspiration pneumonia, the head of the bed should be elevated and the patient watched carefully when he is taking fluids, food, or medications.

Medical treatment—symptoms are treated as they occur. Drug therapy includes the proper anti-infective drug when the causative organism has been identified; oxygen for hypoxemia, but only at the rate of 2 to 3 liters per minute; analgesics as needed for pain; mild hypnotics for sleep; expectorants for cough.

Complications: Empyema, lung abscess, purulent pericarditis, peritonitis, endocarditis, meningitis, arthritis.

Course: Onset is usually abrupt except in atypical (viral) pneumonia, when it may be insidious. Atypical pneumonia is self-limited.

Pneumoconiosis

Other Names: Coal-miner's disease, black lung, silicosis.

Condition: Air sacs of the lungs become filled with an irritating material such as coal dust, asbestos fiber, glass fiber, or silicon, which may cause irritation and prevent air from entering the alveoli.

Treatment: Palliative and supportive.

Prevention: Protection of workers from various industrial dusts that cause the condition.

Pulmonary Infarction (Pulmonary embolism)

Condition: Blockage of an artery or arteriole that supplies blood to a portion of the lung. The size of the vessel affected determines the degree of infarction.

Causes: Venous thrombosis or embolism (blood or fatty material); myocardial infarction; a complication following surgery.

Symptoms and Signs: Substernal pain; weakness; nausea; dyspnea; hyperpnea; fainting. Auscultatory signs: impairment of resonance, pleural friction rub; rales, distant or absent breath sounds; possibly mild icterus; cyanosis; tenderness over the chest; phlebitis of the legs; fall in blood pressure; dilatation of the cervical veins.

Diagnostic Procedures Usually Ordered: White blood cell count; differential count; sedimentation rate; blood chemistry; electrocardiogram; chest x-ray; lung scan.

Treatment: Encourage patient to keep as active as possible and to breathe deeply even if it causes pain (see Appendix G, Breathing Exercises for Home Use). If confined to bed, he should be moved frequently. Helpful measures include elevating the foot of the bed 6 inches and applying warm, moist packs to the chest.

Medical treatment—anticoagulant therapy, which requires close monitoring, especially if heparin is being used; prothrombin time should be checked frequently. Other treatment, symptomatic.

Complications: Pulmonary edema; pleurisy with effusion; secondary lung infection; lung abscess; cor pulmonale; cardiac failure.

Course: Incomplete infarction clears in 2 to 3 days; complete infarction may not clear for 2 to 3 weeks.

Pulmonary Tuberculosis

Condition: An infectious disease of the lungs, characterized by the formation of tubercles in the lung tissue.

Cause: An organism called *Myobacterium tuberculosis*.

Symptoms and Signs: Early—progressive fatigue; malaise; loss of weight. Later—chills; evening rise in temperature; night sweats; cough; sometimes chest pain, dyspnea, hoarseness. Symptoms may be intermittent with periods of remission and exacerbation. Auscultatory signs: impairment of resonance; decrease or accentuation of breath sounds; rales; friction rub.

Diagnostic Procedures Usually Ordered: Sputum examination (a laryngeal swab or stomach washing may be required); sedimentation rate; tuberculin test (unless known to be positive); chest x-ray.

Treatment: First step is confirmation of the clinical diagnosis by examination of sputum (a guinea pig inoculation is done in doubtful cases); then a sensitivity test to determine best chemotherapeutic agent to be used. In most cases two or three drugs given simultaneously produce better results than a single drug. Principal drugs used are ethambutol, isoniazid, aminosalycylic acid (PAS), and streptomycin. When these drugs are ineffective, or in case of relapse, many other drugs can be and are used. Hospitalization is necessary until the patient is no longer infective (usually 4 to 6 months), but not in a nursing home because of possibility of spreading the disease to others. Bed rest for the first part of hospitalization (usually about 2 months), with gradual return to ambulatory status. Surgery not usually advised for elderly patients.

Complications: Pleurisy with effusion; pneumothorax; empyema; atelectasis; extension of the disease process to other organs; severe impairment of pulmonary function.

Course: Variable, but generally the disease responds to chemo-therapeutic agents quite satisfactorily, and arrest is the rule. Remissions and exacerbations not uncommon.

Rhinitis (acute)

Condition: Acute inflammation of the nasal mucous membranes. May be the only symptom of a common cold or of an associated condition such as pharyngitis.
Causes: Usually, a virus. May be precipitated by inhalation of gases, dusty air, or smog; the ingestion of certain drugs such as potassium iodide; or may be simply part of the common cold syndrome.
Symptoms and Signs: In the early stage, dryness of the nose, eyes, and soft palate; malaise; chills; headache. Later, a watery nasal discharge; nasal obstruction; sneezing; excessive tearing; redness of the affected area.
Treatment: Largely symptomatic. Nasal decongestants; analgesics.
Complications: May progress to sinusitis or bronchitis.
Course: Usually self-limited, lasting a few days unless complications occur.

Rhinitis (allergic)

Other Names: Atopic rhinitis; vasomotor rhinitis; hay fever.
Condition: Inflammation of the nasal mucous membranes caused by an allergic reaction.
Causes: Hypersensitivity of the nasal mucosa to inhaled irritants; emanations from animals; certain foods. Precipitating factors include sudden exposure to cold and psychogenic conditions.
Symptoms and Signs: Sneezing; watery nasal discharge; postnasal drip; a feeling of nasal obstruction; narrowing of the nasal cavities; possibly, nasal polyps and lacrimation (tearing).
Diagnostic Procedures Usually Ordered: Skin sensitivity test; white blood cell and differential counts.
Treatment: Remove the cause, if possible. Antiallergenic therapy may be indicated; otherwise treatment is symptomatic.
Complications: Sinusitis; ulceration of the nasal mucosa; nasal polyps; secondary infection.
Course: Depends on whether the cause can be removed and effectiveness of treatment. Seasonal hay fever can more often be prevented than other forms of allergic rhinitis.

Rhinitis (chronic hypertrophic)

Other Name: Chronic hyperplastic rhinitis.
Condition: Chronic, low-grade inflammation of the nasal mucosa.
Causes: Many, including bacterial infection; allergy; repeated attacks of acute rhinitis; paranasal sinusitis; tobacco smoke, dust, and various other irritating inhalants.
Symptoms and Signs: Nasal obstruction; increased nasal secretions; hypertrophy of the nasal mucosa; enlargement of the inferior and possibly the middle turbinate bones; diminished sense of taste and smell; tinnitus and partial deafness; headache.
Treatment: If possible, removal of the cause when known. Mild nose drops; use of a vaporizer; coating the mucosa with petroleum jelly when the atmosphere is dry.
Complications: Secondary infection; sinusitis; deafness.
Course: Depends on effectiveness of treatment.

Sinusitis (acute and chronic)

Condition: Acute or chronic inflammation of the mucous membrane lining of one or more of the paranasal sinuses. When all of the sinuses are involved, the condition is known as pansinusitis.
Cause: Usually, a viral or bacterial infection of the nasal mucosa which extends into mucosa of the sinuses.
Symptoms and Signs: *In both forms*—nasal discharge; postnasal drip; periorbital edema (especially if the frontal sinuses are affected); transillumination may show a darkening of the affected sinus.
   Acute sinusitis—pain over the affected area; headache; fever; toothache (especially if the maxillary sinuses are involved); anorexia; vertigo; malaise; photophobia.
   Chronic sinusitis—recurrent headache; pain and tenderness over the affected sinus.
Diagnostic Procedures Usually Ordered: White blood cell count; differential count; x-ray of affected sinuses.
Treatment: *Acute sinusitis*—analgesics; sedatives; decongestants; broad-spectrum antibiotics; local heat.
   Chronic sinusitis—When the organism has been identified, a suitable anti-infective agent; concomitant treatment of any accompanying disorder; surgery may be needed to provide adequate drainage of the sinuses.
Complications: Sinusal fistula; suppurative adenitis; bronchopneumonia; osteomyelitis of adjacent bones; retrobulbar abscess; brain abscess; meningitis.

Spontaneous Pneumothorax

Condition: The collapse of a lung due to an opening in the visceral pleura that allows air to enter the pleural space.

Causes: May be secondary to trauma, a penetrating wound, or rupture of a bleb or bulla on the surface of the visceral pleura; bacterial or fungal infection of the lungs; emphysema; fibrosis of the lungs.

Symptoms and Signs: In mild cases, the patient may show no symptoms. Usually, sudden severe pain in the chest, with tachycardia and sometimes shock; lack of motion of the affected side of the chest; decrease of breath sounds on affected side; shift of trachea to unaffected side.

Diagnostic Procedures Usually Ordered: Breathing test for vital capacity; chest x-ray at weekly intervals until the lungs return to normal.

Treatment: Rest is all that is required for mild cases, since the opening is self-sealing. In serious cases, air must be removed from the pleural cavity, usually by insertion of a tube and use of a water trap or Stedman pump. Analgesics for pain and to allay apprehension; cough medications.

Complications: Pleural effusion; tension pneumothorax (increase in positive intrapleural pressure), an emergency that requires removal of air from the pleural cavity.

Course: Onset, abrupt. Response to treatment, variable. Subsequent episodes may require resection of the weakened portion of the lung.

Tonsillitis

Condition: Inflammation of the tonsils; may be acute or chronic.

Cause: A viral or bacterial infection; usually occurs in conjunction with pharyngitis, sinusitis, or some other respiratory infection.

Symptoms and Signs: Chills, fever, headache, sore throat, anorexia, difficulty in swallowing, hoarseness, malaise, pain in the muscles and joints, swelling of neighboring lymph glands.

Treatment: Rest, warm throat irrigations, analgesics, the appropriate antibiotic drug. Surgery is indicated if the tonsils are hypertrophied or if infections recur frequently.

Complications: Peritonsillar abscess, otitis media, mastoiditis, sinusitis, rheumatic fever.

Course: Mild cases subside in a few days; severe cases may last from one to two weeks.

CHAPTER 3

Diseases and Disorders of the Circulatory System

Diseases of the blood and lymph
    The anemias
        Aplastic anemia
        Hemolytic anemia
        Iron-deficiency anemia
        Normocytic, normochromic
          anemia
        Pernicious anemia
    Cryoglobulinemia
    Hodgkin's disease
    Leukemia
        Acute leukemia
        Chronic leukemia
    Lymphosarcoma
    Multiple myeloma
    Myelofibrosis
    Polycythemia vera
    Reticulum cell sarcoma
Diseases of the blood vessels
    Arteriosclerosis
    Atherosclerosis
    Carotid artery syndrome
    Cerebrovascular accident
    Thrombophlebitis
    Varicose veins

Disorders of blood pressure
    Hypertension
    Hypotension
    Syncope
        Carotid sinus syndrome
        Orthostatic hypotension
        Vasopressor syncope
Diseases of the heart
    Angina pectoris
        Ischemic heart disease
    Atrial arrhythmias
    Bacterial endocarditis
    Congestive heart failure
    Heart block
        First, second, and third degree
          block
        Sinoatrial block
    Left heart failure (acute)
    Myocardial infarction (acute)
    Pulmonary heart disease
    Valvular heart disease
        Aortic valvular insufficiency
    Ventricular tachycardia (paroxys-
        mal)

DISEASES OF THE BLOOD AND LYMPH

THE ANEMIAS

Aplastic Anemia

Other Names: Hypoplastic anemia; toxic, paralytic anemia; refractory anemia.
Condition: Failure of the bone marrow to produce enough red blood cells.
Causes: Toxic agent, certain drugs, irradiation, viral hepatitis, severe infection; or the cause may be unknown.
Symptoms and Signs: Fatigue, fever, weakness, dyspnea, pallor, petechiae, tachycardia.
Complications: Hemorrhage, infections, septicemia.
Course: Onset is insidious; outcome is usually fatal.

Hemolytic Anemia

Condition: An anemic condition that is due to intravascular destruction of red blood cells; several forms are recognized.
Cause: Often idiopathic. Possible precipitating factors and conditions: leukemia, lupus erythematosus, acute infections, toxic agents, including certain drugs.
Symptoms and Signs: Backache, chills, cyanosis, fatigue, splenomegaly.
Treatment: Removal of the causative agent; possibly, transfusion; sometimes, corticoid therapy.
Complication: Thrombophlebitis.
Course: Onset, gradual. Chronic course with outcome depending on type of anemia and response to treatment.

Iron-Deficiency Anemia

Other Names: Chronic anemia, hypochromic anemia, microcytic anemia, chlorosis.
Condition: A form of anemia in which the red blood cells are smaller than normal and there is a relative or absolute iron deficiency.
Causes: Malnutrition; impaired absorption of iron. In the elderly, a frequent cause is chronic bleeding, especially from the gastrointestinal tract.

Symptoms and Signs: Varied, often not indicative of any specific disorder: weakness, headache, dyspnea, numbness of extremities, pain in the tongue and difficulty in swallowing, appearance of white plaques on the skin, brittle fingernails, slight edema of the feet, systolic murmur, enlargement of the heart and liver.

Diagnostic Procedures Usually Ordered: Complete blood count, stool examination for occult blood, gastrointestinal x-ray series, iron binding and iron serum tests.

Treatment: Remove the cause, if possible.

Medical treatment—administration of iron orally or possibly intramuscularly for at least 3 to 5 months to restore the iron reserve and meet immediate needs. A special technique is required for intramuscular administration to prevent leakage and staining of the skin. The intravenous route is used only in severe conditions; it requires the use of a special preparation of iron.

Side effects of iron therapy—numerous, including gastric irritation and constipation, with black, pasty stools. Both these side effects can be overcome by giving the iron orally with food and by increasing intake of laxative foods. Skin rash and conjunctivitis may occur as delayed side effects; both usually respond to treatment with antihistamines.

Complication: Gastritis.

Course: Depends on patient's response to iron therapy and whether the basic cause can be eliminated.

Normocytic, Normochromic Anemia

Condition: This type of anemia occurs in two forms: (1) that which results from rapid severe loss of blood or rapid destruction of red blood cells; (2) that which results from slow, gradual loss or destruction of red blood cells, or failure of the cells to be produced in required quantities.

Causes: *Type 1*—hemorrhage or rapid destruction of the blood cells.

Type 2—disruption in the normal formation of red blood cells in the bone marrow, infectious diseases such as bacterial endocarditis or rheumatoid arthritis, chronic kidney or liver disease, malignancy, endocrine deficiency, slow loss of blood.

Symptoms and Signs: *Type 1*—weakness, restlessness, air hunger, thirst, nausea, sweating, headache, fainting, rapid shallow respirations, thready pulse, fall in blood pressure.

Type 2—symptoms of the underlying condition, fatigue, anorexia, irritability, pallor, edema, bone tenderness, functional cardiac murmur; possibly, tachycardia, cardiomegaly, hypotension.

Diagnostic Procedures Usually Ordered: *Type 1*—complete blood count, blood chemistry.

Type 2—bone marrow analysis, kidney function tests.

Treatment: *Type 1*—Remove underlying cause, if possible; transfusion of whole blood or packed red cells as soon as the bleeding has stopped.

Type 2—Treat the underlying cause, transfusion when blood loss is severe, institute measures to improve patient's general health.

Complications: *Type 1*—possibly hypovolemic shock when the condition is due to loss of blood volume.

Type 2—markedly lowered resistance to infection.

Course: *Type 1*—depends on the cause of the blood loss and response of the patient to replacement therapy with blood or cells.

Type 2—Onset is insidious; not often serious unless accompanied by kidney disorders.

Pernicious Anemia

Condition: An anemic condition rarely seen in the elderly except as the persistence of an earlier anemia; characterized by poor absorption of vitamin B_{12} from the gastrointestinal tract.

Causes: Possibly a familial trait; lack of secretion of intrinsic factor by the gastric mucosa; poor dietary habits.

Symptoms and Signs: Anorexia, diarrhea, sore tongue, general weakness, dyspnea, anginal pain, tachycardia, pallor or yellowness of skin, enlarged spleen and liver.

Diagnostic Procedures Usually Ordered: Complete blood count; blood cell studies; platelet count; urinalysis with uribilinogen determination; stool analysis; gastric analysis; Shilling test for vitamin B_{12} absorption; bone marrow examination; x-ray of stomach and colon to rule out neoplasm.

Treatment: Improved nutrition; restoration of blood to normal if possible; intramuscular injections of vitamin B_{12}.

Complications: Carcinoma of the stomach, mental deterioration.

Course: Onset is insidious. Improvement may follow dietary therapy and general health measures with restoration of blood to normal.

CRYOGLOBULINEMIA

Condition: Precipitation of certain blood elements in the peripheral vessels. Rarely seen in the elderly.
Cause: Abnormal lowering of the body temperature due to lowering of the temperature of the blood. Basic cause unknown.
Treatment: Measures to keep the patient warm.

HODGKIN'S DISEASE

Other Names: Hodgkin's granuloma; Hodgkin's sarcoma; Hodgkin's parasarcoma. (All are similar to but not identical to Hodgkin's disease.)
Condition: Malignancy of the lymph nodes.
Cause: May be no apparent cause. May possibly be due to infections, granuloma, or neoplastic disease elsewhere in the body.
Symptoms and Signs: Various, according to the particular subdivision of the disease. May include any or all of the following: anorexia; loss of weight; night sweats; pruritus; diarrhea; stridor; pain in the chest; dysphagia; hematuria; paresthesia; pain in the bones (if involved); tachycardia. Later signs—enlargement of the lymph nodes, which are matted and fixed; tenderness over the sternum; continuous or intermittent fever; enlargement of the spleen or liver.
Diagnostic Procedures Usually Ordered: Complete blood count; uric acid test; nodal biopsy.
Treatment: When diagnosed early, radiation to the affected glands may help or even cure; early surgical removal of affected nodes may delay progress of the disease; antineoplastic chemotherapy is sometimes effective. Later treatment: chiefly palliative.
Complications: Intercurrent conditions such as tuberculosis; herpes zoster; hypersplenism; leukemia; or amyloidosis.
Course: Progressive and ultimately fatal unless early treatment is successful.

LEUKEMIA

Acute Leukemia

Other Names: Acute lymphoblastic leukemia, acute myeloblastic leukemia, acute monoblastic leukemia.

Condition: In all forms, an abnormal increase in the number of white blood cells manufactured by the body.

Cause: Usually unknown; possibly a virus in some cases. Possible predisposing factors: chronic benzol poisoning, ionizing radiation, genetic elements.

Symptoms and Signs: Variable. Early symptoms: excessive bleeding (especially after tooth extraction), weakness, fatigue, nosebleed, oral bleeding, pain in the bones and joints, possibly nausea, vomiting, cough, dyspnea, pallor, fetid breath, loss of weight, petechiae, fever. Later symptoms: bone tenderness and enlargement of spleen, liver, and lymph glands.

Diagnostic Procedures Usually Ordered: Complete blood count, x-ray of long bones, examination of aspirated bone marrow.

Treatment: Chiefly palliative and supportive; possibly, blood transfusion to treat the anemia and the low platelet count; ample fluids.

   Medical treatment—Corticosteroids if the white cell count is rising rapidly; analgesics as indicated; oral antibiotics to help prevent infections. An antimetabolite or similar drug may be given unless side effects are serious—should be discontinued when the white blood cell count is reduced to about 10,000.

Complications: Intercurrent infections, intercranial hemorrhage, rupture of the spleen, gastrointestinal ulceration.

Course: Remissions and exacerbations may occur. Usually progressive, with death occurring within 5 to 6 months.

   Chronic Leukemia

Other Names: Chronic lymphoblastic leukemia, chronic myeloblastic leukemia.

Condition: In all forms, a marked increase in the white blood cell count (in the lymphocytic form the lymphocytes predominate; in the myelocytic form the myelocytes predominate).

Cause: Usually unknown. May follow ionizing radiation or exposure to chemical agents such as benzol.

Symptoms and Signs: In both forms, few symptoms in the early stages. Later symptoms: anorexia; flatulence; abdominal pain; diarrhea; occasionally, gastrointestinal bleeding; possibly, enlargement of the spleen.

   Lymphocytic form—first sign may be enlargement of lymph nodes. Later signs: pulmonary infiltration; pleural effusion; lesions of the skin such as papules, vesicles, herpes zoster, or exfoliative (scaling) dermatitis.

Myelocytic form—symptoms of genitourinary involvement such as hematuria, lumbar pain; in the female, abnormal menstrual function.

Diagnostic Procedures Usually Ordered: Complete blood count, examination of aspirated bone marrow.

Treatment: None may be needed. Transfusion may be required for marked anemia, bleeding, or rapid rise in white cell count. All other treatment is palliative and supportive.

Medical treatment—antianemic drugs for the anemia, anti-infective drugs for intercurrent infections, corticosteroids to help alleviate symptoms. Chlorambutal or nitrogen mustard may be given, but the side effects are often severe.

Complications: Hemorrhage, infection, uncontrollable visceral involvement, congestive heart failure are all causes of immediate death.

Course: Onset is gradual and insidious. Remissions and exacerbations may occur. Average survival after diagnosis is 2½ to 3½ years; about 50 percent live as long as 5 years.

LYMPHOSARCOMA

Condition: A malignancy characterized by enlargement of multiple lymphatic glands and infiltration of various tissues. Usually occurs in persons between 60 and 80 years of age.

Cause: Unknown.

Treatment: No curative treatment available.

Course: Survival rate is low.

MULTIPLE MYELOMA

Other Names: Kahler's disease, Bence Jones disease.

Condition: A malignant tumor of the bone marrow.

Cause: Unknown.

Symptoms and Signs: Weakness; neuralgic and skeletal pain; loss of weight; oronasal bleeding; palpable swellings on the ribs, skull, sternum, vertebrae, clavicles, scapulae, and pelvic girdle.

Diagnostic Procedures Usually Ordered: Complete blood count; sedimentation rate; analysis of blood proteins; blood chemistry; urinalysis; examination of aspirated bone marrow; x-rays of various bones; test for Bence Jones protein.

Treatment: Chiefly palliative and supportive. Radiotherapy for severe pain.

Medical treatment—cortisone may relieve symptoms in some patients; oral busulfan (Myleran) may retard the malignant process in the bone marrow, but side effects usually preclude its use.

Complications: Spontaneous fractures; infiltration of the myeloma cells; renal insufficiency; primary amyloidosis.

Course: Progressive and ultimately fatal.

MYELOFIBROSIS

Condition: A rather rare blood disease in which the bone marrow is replaced by fibrous tissue.

Cause: Unknown.

Treatment: No known treatment for the anemia that characterizes this disorder.

POLYCYTHEMIA VERA

Condition: A blood disorder in which more than the usual number of red blood cells, which contain more than the usual amount of hemoglobin, are manufactured in the bone marrow. Usually diagnosed and treated early in life, but may recur in later life.

Cause: Unknown.

Symptoms and Signs: Headache; dyspnea; vertigo; intermittent claudication; vomiting; hematemesis.

Diagnostic Procedures Usually Ordered: Complete blood count; hemoglobin; hematocrit; blood cell studies; platelet count; bleeding time; ophthalmoscopy.

Treatment: Radioactive phosphorus; periodic phlebotomy.

Complications: Peptic ulcers; cerebral, gastrointestinal, and nasal hemorrhage; intercurrent infections; cardiac decompensation; intravascular thrombosis.

Course: Onset usually gradual, occasionally catastrophic with gastrointestinal bleeding or myocardial infarction. Survival related to severity of complications; median survival in treated cases 7 to 14 years.

RETICULUM CELL SARCOMA

Other Names: Reticulosarcoma; reticulocytoma; reticulum cell lymphosarcoma; histiocytic lymphoma.

Condition: A proliferating neoplasm of the reticulum cells (cells that contain a fine network of protoplasm, or cells that form a fine network in certain tissues of the body such as nervous tissue, lymph glands, and connective tissue, including blood). Occurs mostly in older people.

Cause: Unknown.

Symptoms and Signs: Local or generalized enlargement of the lymph glands, usually painless, but often the cause of pressure and obstructive phenomena. Progressive fatigue; anorexia; loss of weight; bone pain and tenderness; pruritus; usually, a firm, discrete mass in the abdomen; moderate enlargement of the spleen and liver; fever; pleural effusion; possibly, nodular infiltration of the skin and subcutaneous tissue.

Diagnostic Procedures Usually Ordered: Complete blood count; blood chemistry; urinalysis, especially for calcium; biopsy; x-ray of sternum and other bones.

Treatment: Surgery, if the area involved is limited. In other cases surgery, radiation, and antimetabolitic drugs may be used.

Complications: Disorders of the spleen; anemia.

Course: Usually, widespread rapid dissemination. Survival time— about 2 to 2½ years after diagnosis.

DISEASES OF THE BLOOD VESSELS

ARTERIOSCLEROSIS

Common Name: Hardening of the arteries.

Condition: Thickening and inflammation of the coats of the arteries with narrowing of the lumen and lessening of the elasticity of the muscular coat.

Causes: Possible precipitating factors include old age, abnormal metabolism of fats, diet rich in fats, endocrine imbalance, diabetes mellitus.

Symptoms and Signs: Depend on the area of the body involved. Any organ or regional part of the body that has diminished arterial circulation will suffer degeneration and death of the affected portion if blockage is complete.

Normal blood vessel

Beginning arterio-
sclerosis

Advanced arterio-
sclerosis

**The lumen of the blood
vessel is narrowed in
arteriosclerosis.**

Treatment: Low-fat diet, vasodilator drugs to control the hypertension that usually accompanies arteriosclerosis, treatment directed to
the area of the body involved.

Complications: Various disorders caused by the changes in the arterial blood supply to the organ or part of the body: for instance,
angina pectoris, coronary occlusion, cerebrovascular accident, nephrosclerosis, thrombosis, infarction, gangrene, aneurysm, or retinal disorders.

Arteriosclerotic heart disease—may lead to coronary occlusion
by causing a blockage of one or more of the coronary arteries; incomplete blockage may cause angina pectoris.

Cerebral arteriosclerosis—refer to neuropsychiatric diseases.

Nephrosclerosis (arteriosclerosis of the blood vessels of the kidney)—may lead to kidney failure, partial or complete, with accompanying high blood pressure and retention of waste products in the
blood.

Arteriosclerosis of the peripheral arteries—may lead to impaired
circulation and loss of the extremity due to gangrenous changes.

Course: Depends on the severity of the condition in the area most
involved and the effectiveness of the treatment.

ATHEROSCLEROSIS

Condition: A blood vessel disorder in which plaques form in the
walls of one or more vessels; those commonly affected include the
carotid, cerebral, coronary, and retinal arteries, where the condition
may progress to partial or total blockage of the vessel.

Causes: Possible precipitating factors include a diet rich in saturated fats, a high level of lipids (fats) in the blood serum, hypertension, diabetes mellitus, release of catecholamines, lack of estrogen (in females), obesity, the use of tobacco.

Symptoms: Depend on the area of the body involved; for example, the coronary arteries, cerebral arteries, or peripheral arteries.

Treatment: Surgical treatment may be used; the atherosclerotic vessel is resected and replaced with a substitute from the patient's body or a synthetic material, providing the vessel is amenable to surgery.

Complications and Course: See arteriosclerosis.

CAROTID ARTERY SYNDROME

Condition: Partial or complete occlusion of one of the internal carotid arteries. More common in older persons.

Causes: Usually caused by an atherosclerotic plaque; sometimes by an embolus or thrombus.

Symptoms and Signs: Usually no symptoms in younger persons or those with an intact Circle of Willis. In others: 5- to 30-minute episodes of intermittent, transient hemiplegia; hemianesthesia; monocular blindness; aphasia ("blackout spells"); possibly focal neurologic signs; absent or diminished pulsation of the carotid artery. In cases of partial occlusion, often a bruit can be heard when a stethoscope is placed over the affected artery. There may be personality changes, confusion, memory defects, or even coma.

If the basilar artery or vertebral artery is involved, symptoms usually include vertigo and an unsteady gait.

Diagnostic Procedure Usually Ordered: Angiogram.

Treatment: Surgery to remove the obstruction; possibly endarterectomy with arterial graft.

Complications: Possibly, neurologic deficits, cerebral infarction.

Course: Slowly progressive when caused by atherosclerosis; may be abrupt if caused by an embolism. (See also Cerebrovascular accident.)

CEREBROVASCULAR ACCIDENT

Other Names: Stroke syndrome, apoplexy, cerebral thrombosis, cerebral hemorrhage, ischemia of the brain.

Condition: A portion of the brain is deprived of its normal blood supply. The affected area may be so small that it goes unnoticed, or so massive as to cause almost instant death.

Causes: Atherosclerosis or arteriosclerosis of the cerebral blood vessels; embolism; rupture of a cerebral aneurysm; trauma; sudden hypotension.

Symptoms and Signs: Varied, depending on the part of the brain involved. Usually vertigo, numbness, diplopia, aphasia, confusion, hemiparesis, hemiplegia. Possibly local neurologic deficit, hyperreflexia, absence of superficial reflexes, and coma. Premonitory signs include dizziness, blurred vision, numbness or weakness, giddiness, slowing of the thought processes, minute personality changes.

Diagnostic Procedures Usually Ordered: Complete blood count, blood chemistry, analysis of spinal fluid, angiogram.

Treatment: *Immediate treatment*—determine the amount of movement the patient is capable of; estimate the amount of muscular coordination that remains; determine how clearly the patient is thinking. Usually at this stage a spinal fluid analysis is done.

Early treatment—prevention of contractures by use of bed board and foot board, no pillows under knees or head, turning the patient frequently to avoid pneumonia and decubitus ulcers. Start rehabilitation within the first week (some start it the first day) under the direction of a physiatrist, if possible. Range of motion exercises three times a day is usual; also passive exercises to even paralyzed muscles. Family or friends can be taught to carry out these exercises until the patient can do them without help. Helpful devices such as slings for arms and for raising up in bed should be supplied. Fluid and electrolyte balance must be maintained. Prevention of mental disorientation is important.

Medical treatment—includes drug therapy as indicated, but the response to drugs may differ from what is usual for the particular drug. Depressants are used with caution as they may increase the depression. Stimulants are usually not used early as they may increase the bleeding if hemorrhage is the cause of the condition.

Later treatment—consists primarily of rehabilitation and depends on the patient's condition.

Complications: Severe neurologic deficit; pneumonia; contractures.

Course: Onset may be sudden or gradual. Progression may be rapid or slow. Factors affecting the course include the severity of the disorder, the extent and location of the lesion, and effectiveness of treatment. The outcome may be death, partial recovery, or complete recovery; when the damage is not massive, partial recovery is the usual outcome. Rehabilitation progresses slowly.

THROMBOPHLEBITIS

Condition: Partial or complete occlusion of a vein by a thrombus (blood clot) with secondary inflammation of the vessel; superficial and deep veins of the leg are most commonly involved.
Causes: May be unknown. Possible causative factors: surgical procedures, trauma, pregnancy, aging, debility, long periods of bed rest, obesity, dehydration, anemia, heart failure, venous stasis.
Symptoms and Signs: Sometimes, none. Usually, pain, discomfort, tenderness, redness, and warmth over the affected vein; slight edema; cyanosis or mottling of the extremity; increase in pulse rate. In the acute stage there is pain, swelling, and cyanosis of the affected extremity; pain on dorsiflexion of the leg. The application of the cuff of a blood pressure machine above the calf and inflation to 80-120 mm Hg will elicit severe pain.
Treatment: *Acute stage*—bed rest with the extremity elevated; external heat; anticoagulant therapy if the deep veins are involved or if there is indication of emboli.
  Later and recovery stages—the use of elastic stockings; anticoagulant therapy may be continued.
Prevention: The wearing of support hose by patients with a tendency to thrombophlebitis; if possible, the avoidance of long standing or sitting in one position without exercising the legs; engaging in proper exercises during and after pregnancy and following surgery.
Complications: Venous insufficiency, pulmonary embolism, pulmonary infarction.
Course: Recovery is usual but recurrences are common.

VARICOSE VEINS

Condition: Abnormal dilatation, elongation, and tortuousness of the superficial veins, usually of the lower extremities. Occurs more often in women than men.
Causes: Often unknown. Possible predisposing factors of the primary type: a familial trait, standing in one position for long periods of time, pregnancy. Possible predisposing factors of the secondary type: thrombophlebitis, increase in venous pressure, phlebitic destruction of tissue at the site of an occlusion in a vein.
Symptoms and Signs: Sometimes, none. Possible soreness, burning,

or pruritus in the region of the varicosities, along with general aching or cramping of the leg muscles. The twisted veins may be seen, especially when the patient is standing.

Treatment: Conservative: the use of elastic stockings and frequent elevation of the extremities. Surgery if conservative treatment is ineffective.

Complications: Rupture of the varicose vein; ulceration; thrombosis; increased pigmentation of skin in the area of varicosities; possibly, stasis dermatitis.

Course: Recurrences are common, even after surgical treatment.

DISORDERS OF BLOOD PRESSURE

HYPERTENSION

Common Name: High blood pressure.

Condition: Any rise in blood pressure above the accepted normal, considering the person's age and general condition. The elevation may be observed during both the diastole and systole or it may be more pronounced in either of these two phases of the heartbeat. A marked rise in diastolic pressure is usually considered to be more serious than a comparable rise in systolic pressure, since systolic pressure varies with exercise, position, emotional status, etc. A rapid rise is also considered more serious than a gradual rise, especially in the older patient. More common in women than in men.

Causes: Many; possible causative factors include kidney disorders, endocrine disturbances, hyperactivity of the vasomotor system, emotional instability, obesity, diabetes mellitus, familial tendency.

Symptoms and Signs: Early stages—usually, none. Later stages—headache, fatigue, nervousness, insomnia, possibly dizziness or dyspnea. Advanced stages—tachycardia, cardiomegaly, flushing, retinopathy, papilledema.

Diagnostic Procedures Usually Ordered: Electrocardiogram; other tests depend on the suspected cause of the condition.

Treatment: For the older patient, gradual moderate reduction is usually considered advisable; blood pressure readings should be taken with the patient lying down and standing.

  Medical treatment—diuretics such as the thiazide preparations may be all that is needed to keep the pressure low enough for safety (patients on diuretics should have a diet rich in potassium to avoid electrolyte imbalance); digitalis if the heart is involved; weight reduction if needed; lowering of salt intake; avoidance of coffee, especially late in the day.

Complications: Congestive heart failure, cerebral thrombosis, hemorrhage, retinopathy, nephrosclerosis, epistaxis, menorrhagia, malignant hypertension.

Course: Onset, usually between 30 and 35 years of age, and gradually rising as one becomes older. Rarely fatal unless complications arise.

HYPOTENSION

Common Name: Low blood pressure.

Condition: A systolic blood pressure that is below 100 and a diastolic pressure that is below 70 or 80 in an individual whose blood pressure is usually within the normal expected limits for his age.

Causes: May be unknown; loss of blood volume, cardiac disorders, shock, certain drug effects, certain infections.

Symptoms and Signs: Lowered blood pressure readings, weakness, fatigue, dizziness, blurred vision, fainting upon standing quickly upright (postural hypotension).

Treatment: Treat the cause if possible; check for possible diabetes mellitus, anemia, or hypothyroidism. Bed rest for a few days and then gradual return to ambulatory status. Hypotensive individuals should never rise quickly from a sitting or lying position.

Medical treatment—antihypotensive drugs such as ephedrine or the steroids when the condition is severe or persistent.

Complications: Cerebrovascular accident; coronary ischemia (myocardial infarction, angina pectoris).

Course: Depends on the cause, the severity of the condition, and whether treatment is successful.

SYNCOPE

Syncope, or fainting, is a fairly common occurrence among the elderly. It may happen as the result of certain physiological conditions, as a reaction to emotional stress, or as a symptom of a blood pressure disorder. Three common disorders that are characterized by syncope are carotid sinus syndrome, orthostatic hypotension, and vasopressor syncope. Because of the frequency with which these conditions occur, each will be discussed as a separate entity.

Carotid Sinus Syndrome

Condition: In this disorder, the individual faints when pressure is applied to the carotid sinus. The sinus may be so sensitive that turning the head, wearing a tight collar, or shaving over the area will induce fainting. In fact, fainting may occur without any observable pressure being applied. More common in men than women.
Cause: Probably the development of atheromatous plaques in the opposite sinus or in the basilar artery.
Symptoms and Signs: Fainting, headache, dizziness or vertigo, unilateral paresthesia, visual disturbances, slurring of speech, bradycardia, hypotension, possibly convulsions.
Diagnostic Procedures Usually Ordered: Electroencephalogram, carotid artery angiogram, brain scan.
Treatment: Three types of this disorder are recognized and treated accordingly: (1) the vagal type occurs most commonly in older people and is treated with atropine; (2) the vasomotor type occurs most commonly in younger people, and is treated with ephedrine; (3) the cerebral type, which occurs in both age groups, is the least common type; it does not respond to medical treatment.

Orthostatic Hypotension

Other Name: Postural hypotension.
Condition: Individual faints if he stands up quickly, even though his blood pressure may be normal when he is seated or lying down.
Causes: Many, including diseases of the autonomic nervous system; specific diseases such as tabes dorsalis, diabetes mellitus, Addison's disease, and some febrile diseases; severe blood loss; cardiac disorders; wasting diseases; bilateral sympathectomy (an operation to relieve hypertension); drug reactions.
Symptoms and Signs: In addition to fainting and the signs of the underlying cause, a tendency to feel faint when changing one's position.
Treatment: Therapy is directed to eliminating the underlying cause of the condition. The patient should be instructed to assume the upright position very slowly; this will usually prevent actual fainting.
Complications: Loss of sphincter tonus with involuntary urination and defecation; muscle wasting; cachexia; symptoms of parkinsonism.
Course: Generally slowly progressive over several years with resulting severe invalidism and eventual death.

Vasopressor Syncope

Other Names: Vasovagal syncope, benign or simple fainting.
Condition: The most common type of fainting, characterized by a sudden fall in blood pressure and an abnormally slow pulse rate.
Causes: Severe pain; increased intra-abdominal pressure, such as may result from straining at stool; emotional stress, for example, grief or bereavement.
Symptoms and Signs: *Early symptoms*—weakness, sweating, restlessness, yawning or sighing, epigastric distress, an anxious appearance, pale, cold, moist skin.
    Later symptoms—blurring of vision, dizziness or lightheadedness, fainting; possibly, a mild convulsion.
Diagnostic Procedure Usually Ordered: Electroencephalogram if the attacks recur or if a convulsion has occurred.
Treatment: Placing the patient in a recumbent position may be all that is needed. Inhalation of aromatic spirits of ammonia may help by stimulating respirations and circulation.
Course: Attacks occur irregularly and may last a few seconds or hours.

DISEASES OF THE HEART

ANGINA PECTORIS

Condition: Moderate inadequacy of the coronary circulation which results in characteristic thoracic pain, usually substernal; precipitated chiefly by overexercise, emotional stress, or a heavy meal, especially at night; relieved by vasodilator drugs and rest.
Cause: Atherosclerosis or arteriosclerosis of the coronary vessels, which causes moderate inadequacy of the coronary circulation and leads to relative hypoxia of the myocardial tissue.
Symptoms and Signs: Sudden, acute attacks of precordial pain, which may extend to the left arm or the throat; feeling of tightness or compression in the chest; anxiety. Between attacks the patient is usually anxious, fearing the next episode.
Diagnostic Procedures Usually Ordered: Electrocardiogram; possibly a chest x-ray to estimate the size of the heart; coronary angiography.
Treatment: Weight reduction, if indicated; smoking is discouraged; avoidance of extremes of temperature. The patient is encouraged to

be as active as possible without overexertion, since this may precipitate an attack. Coronary bypass surgery may be indicated.

Medical treatment—nitroglycerin (grains 1/200 to 1/100) or similar vasodilator given sublingually will usually abort an attack; dosage may be repeated every 15 minutes for three doses. If the vasodilator is not effective, patient should be checked for signs of other cardiac conditions. One of the long-acting nitrates or nitrites may help prevent attacks in some patients.

Complications: Myocardial infarction; congestive heart failure.

Course: Usually, recurrence of attacks at regular or irregular intervals with a possible gradual decline in cardiac function leading to complications. Average life expectancy after first attack—5 to 10 years, although some patients live much longer.

Note: One form of angina pectoris is characterized by attacks that occur without any relation to exercise, often coming on in the early morning and waking the patient from sound sleep. This form of angina tends to appear without any warning and to disappear abruptly.

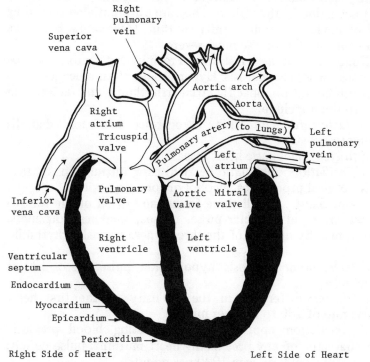

Right Side of Heart   Left Side of Heart

Cross section of heart showing principal divisions, large vessels that enter and leave the heart, and direction of blood flow.

Ischemic Heart Disease

This term may be applied to cardiac disorders in which the blood supply to heart muscle is diminished; it usually refers to angina pectoris or acute myocardial infarction. However, it is not uncommon for an ischemia that cannot be classified as either of these syndromes to occur in older persons. The pain is usually less severe than in anginal episodes in younger persons, but sometimes lasts longer. Physicians consider this ischemia a form of angina rather than a separate disease entity. It may lead to myocardial infarction or congestive heart failure.

ATRIAL ARRHYTHMIAS

**(Including paroxysmal atrial tachycardia,
atrial flutter, and atrial fibrillation)**

Condition: Arrhythmias (alterations in the normal rhythm of the heartbeat) occurring in the atrium. They are differentiated according to degree of deviation from normal rhythm, tachycardia being the least severe and fibrillation the most severe.
Cause: None may be demonstrable. Precipitating factors may be arteriosclerosis or atherosclerosis. Hypertension often precedes or accompanies this condition. Specific atrial arrhythmias and factors that contribute to them include:
   Atrial tachycardia—infection, myocardial infarction, digitalis toxicity, emotional stress.
   Atrial flutter—rheumatic heart disease.
   Atrial fibrillation—rheumatic heart disease, mitral stenosis, thyrotoxicosis, surgical procedures, alcohol or tobacco toxicity.
Symptoms and Signs: In all three forms, any or all of the following: palpitation, rapid irregular pulse, nausea, weakness, dizziness, fainting, dyspnea. Symptoms of the three types of atrial arrhythmias include:
   Atrial tachycardia—cyanosis, hypotension, pulse rate of 100 or more per minute.
   Atrial flutter—difference in the intensity of the first heart sound; pulse rate of 160 to 210 per minute.
   Atrial fibrillation—apprehension; fluctuating blood pressure; change in character of any preexisting heart murmur; pulse deficit; pulse rate of 400 to 600 or even 1000 per minute.
Diagnostic Procedures Usually Ordered: Electrocardiogram; pos-

sibly, circulation time and vital capacity, especially in atrial tachycardia.

Treatment: Atrial tachycardia may be terminated by any one of the following procedures:

1. Apply pressure on the carotid sinus (one side only).
2. Apply gentle pressure on the eyeballs.
3. Instruct the patient to hold his breath and press down on the diaphragm at the same time.
4. Instruct the patient to breathe out against his closed glottis.
5. Induce vomiting.
6. Medication if other measures are ineffective.

Atrial flutter and atrial fibrillation are treated with drugs, usually full digitalization and quinidine, procainamide, or propranolol (Inderal).

Complications: In all three types—embolism. Specific complications include:

Atrial tachycardia—myocardial infarction, congestive heart failure, cardiac necrosis.

Atrial flutter—chronic arrhythmias.

Atrial fibrillation—if prolonged, may cause formation of mural thrombi which may lead to embolism and death.

Course: *Atrial tachycardia*—when uncomplicated, usually responds to treatment. Recurrences are common.

Atrial flutter and fibrillation—see complications listed above. Flutter is less severe than fibrillation.

BACTERIAL ENDOCARDITIS

Condition: Inflammation of the lining of the heart, usually affecting most seriously the endocardium covering the valves. Not often seen in the elderly.

Cause: Usually a gram-positive coccus.

Symptoms and Signs: Chills, sweats, fever, malaise, pain in the joints.

Treatment: The appropriate anti-infective drug. General treatment same as for any severe infection.

Diagnostic Procedures Usually Ordered: Blood culture, sensitivity test.

Complications: Valvular stenosis, cardiac failure. Meningitis and pneumonia are the usual causes of death.

Course: The infection usually responds to treatment. Valvular damage that has occurred cannot be repaired and may cause cardiac insufficiency.

CONGESTIVE HEART FAILURE

Other Names: Cardiac insufficiency, myocardial insufficiency, cardiac decompensation.
Condition: The heart is unable to pump the amount of blood required to meet the metabolic needs of the body.
Causes: Usually occurs as a complication of myocardial infarction, rheumatic heart disease, arteriosclerotic heart disease, or bacterial endocarditis.
Symptoms and Signs: First sign may be dyspnea without exertion. Later—dyspnea even at rest, pain (often in the hepatic area), fatigue, cyanosis, dilation of the neck veins, edema (generalized or pulmonary), ascites. Usually, increased venous pressure, tachycardia, gallop rhythm. Possibly, Cheyne-Stokes breathing, cardiac murmurs, enlargement of liver and spleen.
Diagnostic Procedures Usually Ordered: X-ray of the chest, circulation time, special urinalyses, EKG.
Treatment: Rest in bed and avoidance of any excitement; rotating tourniquets may be used.
  Medical treatment—a quick-acting diuretic to reduce the edema and strain on the heart; anticoagulants if the condition is due to myocardial infarction. Aminophylline or digitalis sometimes ordered.
Complications: Chronic systemic congestion, jaundice, venous thrombosis.
Course: Usually, chronic. Average life expectancy is 5 to 7 years; with treatment, however, 20 years or more is possible.

HEART BLOCK

First, Second, and Third Degree Block

Other Name: Adams-Stokes syndrome.
Condition: Failure of the transfer of some of the atrial impulses to the ventricles (asystole), with resulting slowing of the heart rate, interruption of the heartbeat, or even cardiac standstill. Usually classified as first, second, and third degree heart block.
Causes: Several, including ventricular fibrillation and toxic effects of certain drugs (quinidine, digitalis, Neo-Synephrine, anesthetics);

any condition that disturbs the normal conduction of impulses from the sinoatrial node through the heart.

Symptoms and Signs: Episodes of weakness, accompanied by a rapid fall in cardiac pressure and bradycardia (usually less than 40 beats per minute). Length of the attack determines severity of the symptoms: 4 to 8 seconds—unconsciousness; 12 seconds—pallor, unconsciousness, possibly a few clonic jerks; 5 minutes—all of the above plus cyanosis, stertorous breathing, fixed pupils, incontinence. With resumption of the heartbeat, flushing of the neck and face.

Diagnostic Procedure Usually Ordered: Electrocardiogram.

Treatment: Ephedrine and corticosteroids are sometimes ordered. The patient should avoid undue exercise. Frequent recurrence of the episodes may indicate need for a pacemaker.

Complication: Cardiac failure.

Course: Depends on the severity of the condition and effectiveness of the treatment. Repeated attacks may result in impairment of mental functioning.

Sinoatrial Block

Condition: An interference with the conduction of some of the impulses between the sinus node and the atrioventricular node.

Causes: Toxic effects of certain drugs (digitalis, quinidine, Neo-Synephrine, potassium salts); hyperkalemia; such diseases as diphtheria, pertussis, parotitis. Myocardial ischemia may precipitate an attack.

Symptoms and Signs: Possibly none, or relatively slight signs such as weakness and fainting. Sometimes, prolonged systoles, an irregularly dropped beat, or a missed beat (for example, after every two or three regular beats).

Diagnostic Procedure Usually Ordered: Electroencephalogram.

Treatment: Mild sedation may be all that is needed. Ephedrine is sometimes ordered.

Complication: Prolonged heart block (Adams-Stokes syndrome).

Course: Generally, no prolonged treatment is required. Prognosis is good in most cases.

LEFT HEART FAILURE (ACUTE)

Other Names: Cardiac asthma, nocturnal paroxysmal dyspnea.

Condition: Insufficient cardiac output resulting from functional failure of the left side of the heart.

Causes: Many, including lesions of the aortic or mitral valve; hypertension; coronary sclerosis or thrombosis; sudden increase of the heart load; trapping of blood in the pulmonary vessels.

Symptoms and Signs: Acute attacks occur at night after the patient has had about an hour of sleep. Warning sign—dyspnea on exertion. During the attack—a sense of suffocation, dyspnea, cough (which becomes severe), sweating, wheezing, prolonged expirations, ashen skin, possibly frothy or bloodstained sputum. Auscultatory signs—moist rales, mainly at the base of the lungs; wheezing is heard over all lung fields.

Treatment: Postural drainage (after the emergency is over).

   Medical treatment—early, a strong analgesic to quiet the patient and allay anxiety; possibly oxygen; aminophylline slowly given intravenously. To prevent recurrences, some form of digitalis and possibly a diuretic to help control the congestion.

Complication: Pulmonary edema, of varying degree.

Course: Depends on effectiveness of the treatment and the amount of cardiac reserve the patient has.

MYOCARDIAL INFARCTION

Other Name: Coronary thrombosis.

Condition: A portion of the heart muscle is destroyed due to ischemia (localized tissue anemia) of the area following blockage of a coronary artery, or one of its branches, by either a thrombus or an atherosclerotic condition.

Causes: May develop suddenly, without any history of heart disorder. May also be secondary to arteriosclerotic heart disease; may follow angina pectoris, other heart diseases, or any long-standing disease.

Symptoms and Signs: Severe, crushing, substernal pain, and any or all of the following: cold sweating, nausea, vomiting, dyspnea, shock, anxiety, fever, rales, tachycardia, irregular pulse, gallop rhythm, hypotension.

Diagnostic Procedures Usually Ordered: Electrocardiogram, complete blood count, blood electrolyte and enzyme estimations, sedimentation rate.

Treatment: Usually, bed rest for from 10 to 14 days in a partly raised position (Fowler's). Use of a bedside commode instead of a bedpan helps avoid straining at stool, which should be prevented. Fluid intake and output is monitored to determine renal efficiency.

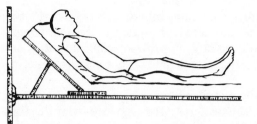

Fowler's Position

Liquid diet at first; soft foods are added gradually as tolerated; salt is usually withheld. Coronary bypass surgery may be indicated.

Medical treatment—vasodilator drugs may not be effective. Anticoagulant therapy may be used, but may be inadvisable for the elderly. Corticosteroid therapy or norepinephrine may be helpful, and oxygen may be used. Constipation is treated with bulk laxatives, fecal softeners, or oily laxatives, as seems best for the patient.

Complications: Shock, pulmonary embolism, atrial embolism caused by mural thrombus, acute pulmonary edema, cardiac aneurysm, arrhythmias, cardiac failure.

Course: Mortality at first attack, 5 to 10 percent. Recurrence is common.

PULMONARY HEART DISEASE

Other Names: Cor pulmonale, right heart failure.

Condition: Enlargement of the right ventricle and eventual heart failure resulting from various pulmonary and vascular disorders. Seen in three forms: subacute, acute, and chronic.

Causes: Usually multiple. In the elderly, common causes include: pulmonary emphysema, increase in pulmonary arterial pressure, pulmonary fibrosis, chronic bronchitis, bronchiectasis, pulmonary tuberculosis, kyphoscoliosis, passive congestion of the lungs, pulmonary thrombosis or embolism.

Symptoms and Signs: Pain and substernal discomfort, cough, expectoration, dyspnea, wheezing, cyanosis, peripheral edema. Possibly, pleural effusion, hepatomegaly, elevation of venous blood pressure, increase in the intensity of the second heart sound.

Diagnostic Procedures Usually Ordered: X-ray of the chest, electrocardiogram, complete blood count, estimation of arterial oxygen and carbon dioxide (arterial blood gases).

Treatment: Removal of the cause, if possible.

Medical treatment—appropriate anti-infective drugs to rid the lungs of infection; oxygen as indicated; diuretics to reduce edema (electrolyte balance must be carefully monitored when diuretics are used); aminophylline during the attack and also to prevent recurrence.

Complication: Congestive heart failure.

Course: In the acute form, the prognosis for recovery from the first attack is good. The chronic form is characterized by recurring episodes, often complicated by respiratory complications; final outcome depends on effectiveness of the treatment and the possibility of ridding the lung of the disorder that precipitated the condition.

VALVULAR HEART DISEASE

Other Names: Valvular stenosis, valvular insufficiency.

Condition: Interference with normal functioning of any one of the heart valves because of stenosis, vegetative infection, or other pathological condition. In the elderly the aortic valve is most often affected when there is no history of previous valvular pathology.

Aortic Valvular Insufficiency

Other Name: Aortic valve regurgitation or incompetence.

Causes: Many. Most commonly, rheumatic heart disease, subacute bacterial endocarditis, syphilis, trauma, dissecting aneurysm of the aorta.

Symptoms and Signs: May exist for a long time with no signs, the condition being revealed only on physical examination. Weakness, lethargy, exertional dyspnea, orthopnea, anginal pain, elevated pulse pressure, visible arterial pulsations, Corrigan pulse. Auscultatory signs include: a heaving apex beat, displaced to the left and lower than normal; high-pitched diastolic murmur; a blowing decrescendo sound at the second or third interspace to the right of the sternum, or at the third or fourth interspace left of the sternum.

Diagnostic Procedures Usually Ordered: X-ray, electrocardiogram, angiogram.

Treatment: Anticoagulant therapy if blood clots are evident or suspected. Young patients whose condition warrants it are treated surgically, but this is not recommended for elderly patients.

Complications: Congestive heart failure.

Course: Depends on extent of damage to the valve and effectiveness of the treatment.

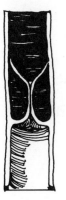 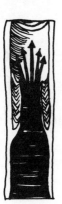

Diagram showing normal action of valves to prevent backflow of blood in veins.

VENTRICULAR TACHYCARDIA (PAROXYSMAL)

Condition: A serious arrhythmia in which heartbeat impulses arise in the ventricles at a rapid rate.

Causes: Most often occurs after severe myocardial infarction or long-standing arteriosclerotic heart disease. Occasionally, occurs after rheumatic valvular heart disease or digitalis toxicity.

Symptoms and Signs: Usually, severe precordial pain of sudden onset; rapid, somewhat irregular pulse; variation in the intensity of the first cardiac sounds; an atrial contraction rate that is lower than the apical beat.

Diagnostic Procedure Usually Ordered: Electrocardiogram.

Treatment: The patient should not use tobacco, tea, or coffee (decaffeinated coffee may be allowed) and should have no heavy meals, particularly in the evening. Carotid sinus pressure is not effective in relieving symptoms.

Medical treatment—Quinidine or procainamide hydrochloride (Pronestyl).

Complication and Course: Ventricular fibrillation is the common complication, may lead to sudden death.

CHAPTER 4

Diseases and Disorders of the Musculoskeletal System

Abnormal spinal curvatures
   Lordosis
   Kyphosis
   Scoliosis
Arthritis
   Acute infectious arthritis
   Rheumatoid arthritis
   Traumatic arthritis
Backache
Bursitis
Cervical Spondylitis
Fibrositis
Fractures
   Compression fracture of the spine

Gout
Hernia
   Femoral hernia
   Herniated intervertebral disc
   Incisional hernia
   Inguinal hernia
   Irreducible hernia
   Obturator hernia
   Umbilical hernia
Osteitis deformans
Osteoarthritis
Osteomalacia
Osteoporosis
Pseudo-gout

ABNORMAL SPINAL CURVATURES

Lordosis

Common Name: Swayback.
Condition: An abnormal increase in the concavity of the spine in the lumbar region; not usually disabling.
Causes: In such cases as pregnancy, severe ascites, abdominal tumor, or kyphosis, lordosis may be compensatory.
Symptoms and Signs: Backache, sometimes.

Kyphosis

Common Names: Hunchback, humpback.
Condition: An abnormal increase in the convexity of the spine in the thoracic region.
Causes: Congenital anomaly, trauma, tuberculosis, poliomyelitis, osteochondrosis of the thoracic vertebrae; sometimes cause is unknown.
Complications: Pulmonary or cardiac disorders, due to the decrease in size and change in shape of the chest cavity.

Scoliosis

Condition: Lateral curvature of the spine; may be to the right or

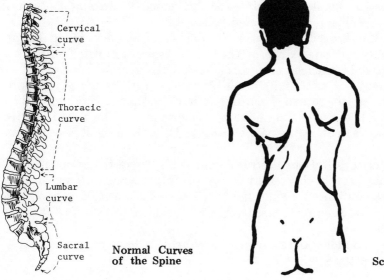

Cervical curve

Thoracic curve

Lumbar curve

Sacral curve

Normal Curves of the Spine

Scoliosis

left, or both (for example, curvature of the thoracic spine to the left and of the lumbar spine to the right).

Causes: Often congenital; may be developmental.

Symptoms and Signs: May be none unless the curvature is marked; hence, the condition may be overlooked. Severe curvature may result in enough pressure on the viscera to cause various disorders.

Treatment: Braces or other support, exercise to develop and strengthen muscular control of the spine.

Course: If congenital or developmental scoliosis is not corrected before the bone structures are "fixed," the condition becomes permanent. Untreated, the condition may lead to visceral disorders in later years.

ARTHRITIS

Acute Infectious Arthritis

Other Names: Pyogenic arthritis; suppurative arthritis.

Condition: An infection of one or more joints by a pyogenic organism; most commonly affects the wrists and weight-bearing joints.

Cause: A pyogenic bacterium, usually gonococcus, meningococcus, staphylococcus, streptococcus, or pneumococcus. Predisposing factors include trauma, intra-articular injections, bacteremia.

Symptoms and Signs: Pain that increases with movement; swelling and heat in the affected joint, and thickening of surrounding tissues; anorexia; chills; fever; increased pulse rate.

Diagnostic Procedures Usually Ordered: Complete blood count; sedimentation rate; x-ray of the joints; aspiration of joint fluid for analysis and for smear, culture, and sensitivity tests.

Treatment: Until results of culture and sensitivity tests are reported, one of the broad-spectrum antibiotics. Later, the appropriate anti-infective drug, and incision and drainage, if indicated. Active exercises as soon as the pain will allow. Other treatment is symptomatic.

Complications: Bone destruction or stiffening of the joints, if treatment has been inadequate. For chronic infectious arthritis characterized by continuous or intermittent low-grade infection and varying intervals between episodes; treatment is similar to that for the acute condition.

Course: Sudden onset. When treatment is prompt and effective, recovery is the rule.

Rheumatoid Arthritis

Other Names: Atrophic arthritis; arthritis deformans.
Condition: Chronic inflammation of the muscles and joints, particularly of the hands, feet, and knees. Two to three times more common in women than in men.
Causes: Unknown. Contributing factors include familial tendency; cold, damp climate; derangement of the immunological mechanism; possibly, hypersensitivity.
Symptoms and Signs: Many and varied. All manifestations are symmetrical and migratory. Pain and stiffness of the hands, feet, and knees, more pronounced in the morning; skin over the extremities is pale, taut, and shiny; anorexia; fatigue; swelling and deformity of the affected joints; muscle atrophy and imbalance; sweating of the palms and soles; firm, painless subcutaneous nodules near the joints; bilateral inflammation of the uvea and conjunctiva of the eye with inadequate flow of tears; pleuritis; splenomegaly; peripheral neuropathy; chronic ulcers of the legs.
Diagnostic Procedures Usually Ordered: Complete blood count, sedimentation rate, serum protein analysis, rheumatoid factor determination, x-rays of the joints.
Treatment: No specific treatment available. Physical therapy for palliation; splinting when there is danger of contractures. Drug therapy is successful in varying degrees; aspirin is commonly used, plus gold salts and corticosteroids. Sometimes surgical replacement of damaged joint surfaces is done to restore function.
Complications: Contractures, joint deformities, loss of function.
Course: Chronic and progressive. Onset usually in the fourth decade, but may occur earlier; often first appears in the spring. Usually only one joint is involved at first, later others. Periods of remission and exacerbation. When symptoms persist for two or three years, cure is seldom complete.

Traumatic Arthritis

Condition: The presence of scar tissue around a joint that has been injured.
Causes: Strain, sprain, dislocation, or fracture of a joint.
Symptoms and Signs: Pain, swelling, and limitation of movement in the affected joint.
Diagnostic Procedure Usually Ordered: X-ray.
Treatment: Emergency treatment—immobilization and the applica-

tion of ice packs to the joint to reduce swelling and bleeding (unless contraindicated by other injuries). Later treatment—after 24 to 72 hours, local heat to reduce pain and increase circulation and healing; important for the joint not to bear any weight if a lower extremity is involved.

Complication: Limitation of movement of the joint.

Course: Recovery is the rule, but in older persons this takes longer and there is more likelihood of residual impairment of function.

BACKACHE

Condition: Aching pain anywhere along the course of the spine; the lumbar region is most apt to be affected.

Causes: May accompany many diseases and disorders (gynecological, prostatic, renal, and vertebral disorders; spinal curvatures); use of poor body mechanics; too soft a mattress, or one that prevents proper alignment of the body while sleeping; use of chairs that are too high or too low; improper methods of standing or walking; remaining too long in one position; improperly fitted glasses, which cause one to move the head in abnormal positions in order to see more clearly; pregnancy.

Symptoms and Signs: Pain or discomfort in any area of the back.

Treatment: Removal or treatment of the cause.

BURSITIS

Condition: Inflammation of one or more bursae, most commonly the deep bursae.

Cause: Unknown. May occur as a result of trauma, rheumatoid arthritis, infection, tuberculosis, syphilis, or gout.

Symptoms and Signs: Pain, swelling, tenderness, and various degrees of limitation of motion in the affected bursae; possibly, palpable fibrinous or calcific granules in superficial bursae.

Diagnostic Procedure Usually Ordered: X-ray of the affected area.

Treatment: Local injection of the steroids, physical therapy; sometimes, surgery.

Complications: Infection and/or complete loss of function of the area involved.

Course: Usually progressive; interfering with the function of a major joint. Remissions and exacerbations are characteristic.

CERVICAL SPONDYLITIS

Other Names: Degenerative cervical arthritis; cervical osteoarthritis.
Condition: Localized osteoarthritis of the cervical spine.
Causes: The process of aging, trauma.
Symptoms and Signs: Recurrent pain or discomfort in the neck; stiffness and limitation of movement in the neck, shoulder, arms, or hands; paresthesias of the fingers, one half of the hand, and over the ulna; muscular weakness; unsteady gait. Possibly, numbness of the trunk and extremities; paralysis of the upper extremities; impairment of biceps and triceps reflexes; kyphosis of the upper thorax. The neck is held in an extended position with the seventh cervical vertebra prominent and often covered with a pad of fat.
Diagnostic Procedures Usually Ordered: X-ray of spine, myelogram, spinal fluid analysis.
Treatment: Usually, cervical traction. If traction fails, surgery may be required. Drug therapy includes analgesics and muscle relaxants as indicated.
Complication: Limitation or loss of normal function.
Course: Tends to be chronic and progressive; outlook, guarded.

FIBROSITIS

Other Names: Rheumatism, rheumatoid myositis.
Condition: Inflammation of the fibrous tissues of the body; does not usually involve the joints.
Cause: Unknown. Precipitating factors include long exposure to cold or dampness, and trauma.
Symptoms and Signs: Pain, stiffness, and soreness over various parts of the body.
Treatment: No known cure. Rest, physical therapy, analgesics.
Course: Recurrences are common.

FRACTURES

Condition: A break in the continuity of a bone. As people grow older, their bones contain progressively less organic and more inorganic (mineral) material than those of younger people, hence are more brittle and break easier. Fractures may be traumatic or pathological and may involve any bone; hip fracture is relatively common and serious in the elderly.

Causes: Osteoporosis; also, extra pull on muscles attached to bones that are very brittle.

Symptoms and Signs: Same as for fractures in all age groups.

Treatment: Same as for fractures in all age groups; hip fracture requires orthopedic surgery.

Compression Fracture of the Spine

Other Names: Collapse of vertebrae, wedge vertebral fracture.

Condition: A vertebral fracture in which the body of one or more vertebrae is compressed.

Causes: Neoplasm; trauma such as a flexion injury to the spine, a blow on the head as may occur when diving into shallow water (fracture of cervical vertebrae), or injury as may occur when jumping from a height and landing on one's feet (fracture of thoracic vertebrae).

Symptoms and Signs: Local pain, increased by movement of the spine or by percussion; unilateral or bilateral pain at the root of spinal nerves; weakness of muscles; possibly, numbness of the trunk and extremities, paresis, loss of bladder and/or bowel control. In severe cases, quadriplegia, areflexia, partial or complete sensory impairment, pathological reflexes. Symptoms of pressure on viscera may result from the change in contour of the spine.

Diagnostic Procedure Usually Ordered: X-ray of the spine.

Treatment: Depends on age and condition of the patient, number of vertebrae involved, and whether there is pressure on the spinal cord or nerves. Symptomatic treatment includes analgesics as needed for pain, local application of heat, mechanical supports of various kinds, surgery if other measures are not effective in relieving symptoms.

Complications: Permanent neurological deficit.

Course: More apt to occur and to be serious in older patients than in young persons because of the degenerative changes that occur in the bones. Course is slow and discouraging. Final outcome depends on extent of the injury and effectiveness of treatment.

GOUT

Condition: An inborn error of metabolism characterized by excessive retention of urates in the blood with deposition in joints (usually unilateral), most commonly in the metatarsal-phalangeal joint of the great toe and in subcutaneous tissue. May occur at any age but often begins in the fourth decade of life. More common in men than in women.

Causes: Basic cause unknown. Predisposing factor: a diet high in purines.

Symptoms and Signs: Pain, swelling, redness, tenderness of affected joints; tense shiny skin over affected joints; limitation of motion. Tophi may appear anywhere in the body but most often in the joints and in the ear lobes.

Diagnostic Procedures Usually Ordered: Sedimentation rate; complete urinalysis including uric acid determination.

Treatment: Allopurinol, colchicine, and probenecid during acute attacks; probenecid between attacks to aid in prevention.

Complications: Chronic gout with degeneration of joints, renal disorders due to urate deposits.

Course: Chronic, with remissions and exacerbations.

HERNIA

A hernia is an abnormal protrusion of an organ or part of an organ through a weakened area in the structures that normally contain it.

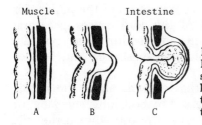

Formation of Intestinal Hernia.   A normal structure;   B   simple hernia;   C   strangulation of loop of intestine.

Femoral Hernia

Condition: Protrusion of a part of the intestine through a weak place in the femoral ring. More common in women than in men.

Causes: Congenital weakness, increased intra-abdominal pressure due to obesity or pregnancy.

Symptoms and Signs: Usually, a painless swelling that persists even when the patient is lying down; a palpable mass below the inguinal ligament.

Treatment: Surgery if feasible. Otherwise, some mechanical means of holding the intestine within the abdominal cavity is used, usually a truss.

Complication: Incarceration of a portion of the bowel.

Course: Outcome depends on effectiveness of treatment and whether incarceration occurs.

Herniated Intervertebral Disc

Other Names: Discogenic disease; ruptured intervertebral disc; herniated nucleus pulposus; protrusion of intervertebral disc; traumatic discopathy.

Condition: Rupture and protrusion of a portion of one or more intervertebral discs into the spinal canal, often causing pressure on the spinal nerve roots that results in severe pain. May occur in any area: approximately 10 percent of all cases occur in the cervical area and 90 percent in the lumbar area.

Causes: Trauma (sudden twisting or straining); lifting too heavy an object, especially if in an unusual position.

Symptoms and Signs: *Cervical disc involvement*—unilateral or bilateral pain, sometimes continuous, more often paroxysmal, which radiates from the area of the lesion to the arms and fingers and is increased by coughing, sneezing, or straining; paresthesia of fingers; weakness or atrophy of biceps or triceps muscle; restriction of neck motion. If the herniation is central and anterior, symptoms of spinal cord involvement may occur (excessive contraction of the pupils, for example). Damage to the lateral half of the cord causes ipsilateral motor paralysis; loss of vibratory, joint, and tendon sensations; decreased tactile discrimination; contralateral anesthesia and loss of temperature sense.

Lumbar disc involvement—pain that extends along the sciatic nerve to the calf and ankle and is increased by coughing, sneezing, or straining; straightening of the spinal curve; scoliosis toward the side opposite the pain; limitation of motion on the affected side; tenderness over the affected area; some weakness of the foot and decreased or absent ankle jerk; paresthesia; limping; rarely, loss of bladder control.

Diagnostic Procedures Usually Ordered: Myelogram and x-ray of the spine, analysis of spinal fluid.

Treatment: *Cervical disc involvement*—acute stage—bed rest with use of cervical traction. Later stages or mild cases—intermittent use of cervical traction at home, in a clinic, or in doctor's office; use of a collar; local applications of heat, diathermy, or similar measures.

Lumbar disc involvement—acute stage—bed rest with use of a bed board, traction to lower extremities, local heat, analgesics. Later stages—use of a low back brace, belt, or other support; teaching the patient proper body mechanics to avoid a recurrence.

Surgery may be required for either cervical or lumbar disc involvement if conservative measures are not effective in relieving symptoms.

Complications: Damage to spinal cord, bladder or bowel incontinence.

Course: Conservative treatment may effect partial recovery, sufficient for the patient to carry on most activities. Residual motor dysfunction, muscular atrophy, and sensory changes may persist. Surgical repair of the injury usually affords relief from pain and may reverse residual conditions wholly or in part. Outlook better for younger persons than for the elderly.

Hiatal Hernia

See Diseases and Disorders of the Gastrointestinal Tract, page 47.

Incisional Hernia

Other Name: Surgical hernia.

Condition: Protrusion of part of the abdominal contents through the abdominal wall at the site of an incision. Vertical incisions are more prone to herniation than horizontal ones.

Causes: Failure of the muscular and other tissue layers to remain in apposition following surgery. Predisposing factors include wound infection, use of drainage tubes, unduly tight stitches, obesity, poor preoperative nutrition, abdominal distention, severe postoperative coughing.

Symptoms and Signs: Sometimes, severe pain, especially if the hernia is incarcerated. Usually, mild abdominal discomfort; and an irreducible mass can be felt as well as the defect in the abdominal wall.

Treatment: Surgery.

Complications: Intestinal obstruction or strangulated hernia.

Course: Depends on effectiveness of treatment and whether obstruction and/or strangulation occurs.

Inguinal Hernia

Condition: A hernia that protrudes through a weak place in the inguinal ring.
Cause: A part of the intestine becomes surrounded by a sac of peritoneum. When intra-abdominal pressure pushes the sac through a weak place in the abdominal wall, the condition is called a *direct hernia*. When the pressure pushes the sac downward into the inguinal canal, the condition is called an *indirect hernia*. An indirect hernia of long standing, with the viscera fixed in the sac, is called a *sliding hernia*.
Symptoms and Signs: *Direct hernia*—painless swelling in the inguinal region that is reducible when the patient is lying down; a palpable, visible mass protrudes through the posterior wall of the inguinal canal, at times into the scrotum; sometimes, a dragging sensation.
  Indirect hernia—similar to direct hernia except that the visible, palpable mass is apt to be painful; the pain is relieved when the patient lies down.
  Sliding hernia—similar to those for direct and indirect hernia except that the mass is not reducible and is not affected by lying down.
Treatment: Surgery, if feasible. Otherwise, some mechanical means of holding the protruding structures in place is used, usually a truss.
Complications: All types: recurrence, strangulation, or incarceration.
Course: Direct hernia is most often seen in elderly men; outcome depends on whether complications occur and effectiveness of treatment. Indirect hernia is seen most commonly in children and middle-aged men; outcome is the same as for direct hernia. Sliding hernia is a chronic condition of long standing; most commonly seen in adults and older persons; outcome is the same as for direct hernia.

Irreducible Hernia

Other Names: Incarcerated hernia, strangulated hernia.
Condition: A hernia that cannot be reduced manually even when the patient is lying down, a complication that can occur with any hernia but is more apt to occur in some hernias than others. A loop of intestine remains in the hernial sac and is pinched off, usually at the wall structure. Feces may be impacted within the lumen of the intestine in the sac. An incarcerated or strangulated hernia is an

irreducible hernia in which the loop of intestine becomes twisted, thus causing an obstruction.

Symptoms and Signs: Pain, usually severe, in the area of the hernia; nausea; vomiting; constipation; anorexia; abdominal distention; passage of blood-stained mucus; presence of a firm, tender mass that increases in size when the patient is straining, and which cannot be reduced. All features of intestinal obstruction are seen.

Treatment: Emergency surgery.

Complications: Peritonitis, septicemia, or gangrene of the affected bowel if condition is allowed to persist for more than a few hours.

Course: Depends on length of time the hernia has been irreducible, whether a complication occurs, and effectiveness of the treatment.

Obturator Hernia

Condition: A hernia due to weakness in the obturator canal. More common in women, especially older women, than in men.

Cause: A congenitally large obturator canal.

Symptoms and Signs: Intermittent pain along the thigh radiating to the knee (Howship-Romberg sign), abdominal pain and rigidity which increase on movement of the hips, palpable mass that can be felt on rectal examination.

Treatment: Surgery.

Complications: Irreducibility and/or strangulation of the hernia.

Course: Surgical treatment is usually successful.

Umbilical Hernia

Other Names: Exomphalos, omphalocele.

Condition: A hernia at the site of the umbilicus. Although most common in children, umbilical hernia also occurs in adults.

Cause: Congenital defect in the umbilical scar. Possible precipitating factors include intestinal obstruction, chronic severe cough, ascites, pregnancy; possibly, obesity.

Symptoms and Signs: Disorders of the upper gastrointestinal tract and/or intestinal obstruction.

Diagnostic Procedures Usually Ordered: X-ray.

Treatment: Surgery.

Complications: Strangulation or incarceration.

Course: Depends on whether a complication occurs and effectiveness of treatment.

OSTEITIS DEFORMANS

Other Name: Paget's disease.

Condition: A nonmetabolic bone disease characterized by excessive destruction of bone and of the bone formation process with resulting characteristic deformities; usually occurs in persons over 40 years of age.

Cause: Unknown. Possible contributing factors include vascular disease, skeletal stress and strain, and localized diseases that are accompanied by bone destruction.

Symptoms and Signs: May be none. Any or all of the following signs may occur, although they are seldom diagnostic: dull, deep pain, most often in one knee; headache; decreased auditory acuity; kyphosis; pendulous abdomen; waddling gait; enlargement of the cranial vault. Bones most apt to be affected are those subject to the greatest amount of stress. Possibly, bowing of the arms and legs, and flattening of the vertebrae and pelvic bones with resulting loss of stature.

Diagnostic Procedures Usually Ordered: Blood chemistry, urinalysis for hypercalciuria, x-ray of affected area.

Treatment: High protein diet with vitamins C and D added, anabolic hormones or corticosteroids.

Complications: Pathological (spontaneous) fractures, deformities, hypercalcemia, renal calculi, estrogenic sarcoma, cardiac failure.

Course: Chronic and progressive; outlook is unfavorable.

OSTEOARTHRITIS

Other Names: Hypertrophic, degenerative joint disease; hypertrophic arthritis; senescent arthritis.

Condition: Degeneration of articular cartilages and hypertrophy of the marginal articulating portions of the bone.

Cause: Unknown. Contributing causes include the physiological process of aging, repeated trauma, and certain constitutional factors.

Symptoms and Signs: Exercise is accompanied by joint pain that disappears with rest, but rest increases the tendency toward joint stiffness; nodular thickening of the joints; tenderness; crepitation; ankylosis; occasionally, warmth or erythema.

Diagnostic Procedure Usually Ordered: X-rays of the joints.

Treatment: No curative treatment is available. Symptomatic treatment includes rest, heat, analgesics, and weight reduction if the patient is obese.

Complication: Osteoarthritis so severe that limitation of activity becomes quite crippling.
Course: Onset is insidious, course is progressive and chronic.

OSTEOMALACIA

Condition: An adult form of rickets, characterized by a deficiency of calcium and phosphorus in the bones.
Causes: Inadequate intestinal absorption and metabolism of calcium, increase of excretion of calcium by the kidney, decrease of calcium and phosphorus in body fluids. Contributing causes include renal acidosis, steatorrhea, and inadequate deposition of minerals in newly formed bone.
Symptoms and Signs: Pain, tenderness, and aching of the bones; sometimes, deformity of the spine or of the skull, muscular weakness, anorexia, loss of weight, a waddling gait.
Diagnostic Procedures Usually Ordered: Blood chemistry, urinalysis for hypercalciuria, x-rays of the affected areas.
Treatment: Large doses of vitamin D. Other treatment is symptomatic.
Complications: Multiple spontaneous fractures; renal calculi; infections of the urinary tract, such as chronic pyelonephritis.
Course: Usually reversible under appropriate treatment. Involvement of the kidneys may result in cardiac paralysis due to hypercalcemia.

OSTEOPOROSIS

Other Name: Bone degeneration.
Condition: A condition characterized by loss of bone matrix, which leads to thinning of the bones of the skeleton.
Causes: Many, varied, and usually multiple. Decreased osteoblastic activity, insufficient production or rate of formation of matrix of bone, disturbance of the ratio between bone formation and bone absorption, disorder of protein and mucopolysaccharide metabolism, malnutrition, hyperthyroidism, diabetes mellitus, Cushing's syndrome, vitamin C deficiency, senility, eunochoidism, treatment with cortisone.
Symptoms and Signs: Pain in the back and the bones, muscular weakness, renal calculi, spontaneous fractures with deformities.

Diagnostic Procedures Usually Ordered: Blood chemistry, urinalysis for hypercalciuria, x-rays of affected areas.
Treatment: High protein diet with phosphorus supplement, endocrine therapy.
Complications: Spontaneous fractures.
Course: Progressive; may be slowed or halted, but is not reversible.

PSEUDO-GOUT

Other Names: Articular chondrocalcinosis, calcium pyrophosphate disease.
Condition: Similar to gout, except that calcium crystals, not urates, are deposited in the synovial fluid of the joints.
Cause: Unknown.
Symptoms and Signs: Similar to those of gout, except that the joints most often involved are the knees. Leukocytosis is a common symptom.
Diagnostic Procedures Usually Ordered: Complete blood count, aspiration of joint fluid for laboratory examination.
Treatment: Intra-articular injection of a corticosteroid, salicylates, phenylbutazone. Colchicine is not recommended.
Complication: Joint degeneration.
Course: Chronic, with remissions and exacerbations.

CHAPTER 5

Endocrine and Nutritional Disorders

The several diseases and disorders described in this section rarely begin in old age. However, many if not most of them are chronic conditions that may very well carry over into the later years of life.

ADRENOCORTICAL HYPERFUNCTION

Other Name: Cushing's syndrome.
Condition: A chronic disorder of the adrenal cortex characterized by excessive secretion of the glucocorticoid hormones.
Causes: Hyperplasia, adenoma, or carcinoma of the adrenal cortex; or may be iatrogenic resulting from administration of cortisone or its derivatives over long periods of time.
Signs and Symptoms: Many and varied. "Moon-face," plethoric appearance, weakness, and fatty deposits especially around the trunk, are outstanding.
Diagnostic Procedures Usually Ordered: Many. Specific urine tests; complete and differential blood count; pyelogram; x-rays of pelvis, spine, skull.
Treatment: Surgical.
Complications: Diabetes mellitus; increased susceptibility to infections; pathological fractures; vascular accidents.
Course: Chronic, with remissions and exacerbations.

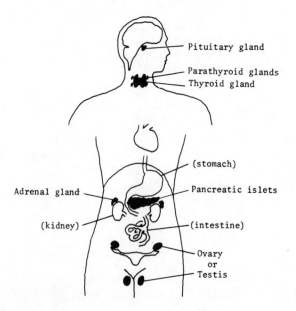

Pituitary gland
Parathyroid glands
Thyroid gland

(stomach)
Adrenal gland
Pancreatic islets
(kidney)
(intestine)
Ovary
or
Testis

The Endocrine System

ADRENOCORTICAL HYPOFUNCTION

Other Name: Addison's disease.
Condition: A disorder that results from inadequate secretion of the adrenal cortex hormone.
Causes: Many possible causes including idiopathic atrophy; amyloidosis; tuberculosis; leukemic infiltration; syphilis; and tumors.
Symptoms and Signs: Many and varied. Severe general weakness and excessive pigmentation of the skin are most common.
Diagnostic Procedures Usually Ordered: Various, including water excretion and salt deprivation tests; electrocardiogram; electroencephalogram.
Treatment: Removal of the cause, if known. Otherwise, treatment includes general health measures; correction of electrolyte imbalance; administration of hormones, with dosages always individualized; blood transfusions; hydrocortisone.
Complication: Gastric irritation sometimes.
Course: Favorable with treatment (glucocorticoids, mineralocorticoids, androgens). Patients should carry identification cards indicating illness and cortisone treatment.

ADRENOGENITAL SYNDROME

Condition: Malfunctioning of the adrenal cortex with resulting changes in the sexual qualities and attitudes of the individual.
Causes: Usually, hyperplasia or neoplasm of the adrenal cortex.
Symptoms and Signs: Vary with the sexes: In the female: oligomenorrhea or amenorrhea (if menopausal), deepening of the voice, hirsutism, and various other signs denoting a tendency toward masculinity including changes in the breasts, genitalia, and skin. In the male: infertility and reduction in the size of the testes.
Diagnostic Procedures Usually Ordered: Urinalysis; possibly, tomography.
Treatment: Surgery and/or replacement hormone therapy.
Complication: Possible progression to malignancy.
Course: With surgery, outcome favorable.

ALDOSTERONISM (PRIMARY)

Condition: A relatively uncommon disorder characterized by electrolyte disequilibrium resulting from excessive production of aldo-

sterone by the adrenal gland; occurs more often in women than men.
Cause: Tumor of the adrenal medulla.
Symptoms and Signs: Episodes of severe headache, tachycardia,
and/or palpitation; nausea; vomiting; polyuria; hyperkalemia; anginal
type pain; aphasia; abdominal pain; hypertension; and/or loss of consciousness. Postural change, exertion, or stress may precipitate an
attack.
Diagnostic Procedures Usually Ordered: Urinalysis, blood chemistry, x-ray, electrocardiogram.
Treatment: Surgery, with replacement therapy that is individually
adjusted.
Complications: Hypokalemia; degeneration of kidney tubules; degeneration of skeletal muscle.
Course: Outlook favorable after removal of the tumor.

AMYLOIDOSIS

Condition: The deposition of amyloid (a proteinaceous polysaccharide substance) in various tissues of the body, usually occurring after
age 40.
Causes: Principal cause thought to be a deficiency or failure to
utilize vitamin C. Often associated with or follows such debilitating
diseases as tuberculosis, chronic arthritis, chronic osteomyelitis, pulmonary abscess or malignancy, multiple myeloma, or disturbance of
endogenous metabolism. Primary amyloidosis may be due to a familial trait.
Symptoms and Signs: Vary greatly and often are not diagnostic.
   Primary amyloidosis—difficulty in breathing, swallowing, and
enunciating words; joint pain; muscle weakness; hypertension; enlarged tongue; yellowish plaques on mucous membranes of the
mouth; extravasation of blood into skin of the face, especially
around the eyes; loss of weight; edema; disorders of the lymph
glands; nervous disorders.
   Secondary amyloidosis—vary according to the primary disease
and/or the organs affected. Usually hypertension, edema, ascites, enlargement of the liver and/or spleen. With infiltration into the mucous membrane of the duodenum and jejunum, malabsorption syndrome may occur. Infiltration into the myocardium usually results in
symptoms of congestive heart failure.
Diagnostic Procedures Usually Ordered: *Primary amyloidosis*—
blood chemistry, tissue biopsy.

Secondary amyloidosis—urinalysis, blood chemistry, sulfobromophthalein test.

Treatment: Treatment of the primary or causative condition may consist of giving vitamin C, but this may be more important in preventing than curing since irreparable damage to the tissues may have occurred. If the amyloid deposits are concentrated in one or a small number of "tumors," they may be excised. Corticoid therapy has been beneficial in some cases.

Complications: Splenomegaly; hepatomegaly; kidney complications; congestive heart failure; hemolytic anemia.

Course: Onset is often insidious. Progressive course unless treatment of attending complications is effective. Death usually occurs within one to three years after onset.

BERIBERI

Other Names: Endemic polyneuritis, burning feet syndrome.

Condition: An endemic nutritional disorder that occurs chiefly in persons whose diet consists almost exclusively of white (polished) rice; characterized by extreme debility.

Causes: Diet that is deficient in vitamin B_1 (thiamine) and perhaps other vitamins; possibly, protein starvation and/or the inability to assimilate thiamine.

Symptoms and Signs: Depend on the severity of the deficiency. Early, the condition may be asymptomatic. Although first symptoms are varied and multiple, they may not be diagnostic. Later, numbness, tingling, muscle tenderness and atrophy beginning in the extremities; sometimes, blindness, respiratory dysfunction due to involvement of the phrenic nerve, cardiac dysfunction, generalized edema, neurologic symptoms.

Diagnostic Procedures Usually Ordered: Blood chemistry, urinalysis, x-ray (especially of the right side of the heart).

Treatment: Primarily dietary consisting of a well-rounded diet plus supplementary vitamin B_1 and other vitamins of the B complex. General health measures.

Complications: Cardiac symptoms. If untreated, incapacitation and eventual death.

Course: Recovery is the rule unless irreparable damage has been done to structures and tissues.

CACHEXIA

Condition: A symptom, not a disease entity; characterized by malnutrition, emaciation, and debility.

Cause: May result from or be concomitant with such diseases and disorders as hypopituitarism, Hodgkin's disease, most forms of cancer, malaria, myxedema, malabsorption syndrome, and any other disorder that produces malnutrition, emaciation, and debility.

Symptoms and Signs: In addition to those stated above, a grayish color to the skin; lusterless hair; dull expression in the eyes; and loss of muscle tone and mass.

Diagnostic Procedures Usually Ordered, Treatment, Complications, and Course: Depend upon the underlying condition.

CARCINOMA OF THE THYROID

Condition: A malignant tumor of the thyroid gland; several types are recognized. More common in women than in men.

Cause: Unknown. Some forms possibly precipitated by irradiation of the head and neck, or by a preexisting benign adenoma of the thyroid or goiter.

Symptoms and Signs: Some forms may be asymptomatic until they press upon adjacent structures. Possible symptoms include hoarseness, cough, difficulty in swallowing, loss of weight, pain in the bones and pathological (spontaneous) fractures, enlargement and hardening of the gland, a palpable nodule in a lobe of the gland.

Diagnostic Procedures Usually Ordered: Uptake of iodine[125] or iodine[131]; x-ray.

Treatment: Surgery, irradiation, thyroid-suppressant drugs.

Complications: Spread to adjacent structures, especially the cervical lymph glands.

Course: Prognosis is guarded; varies with the type of tumor. When surgical excision is complete, the prognosis is good.

DERMATOMYOSITIS

Condition: A noninflammatory, sometimes fulminating disorder affecting mainly the skin and striated muscle tissues, and often associated with malignant neoplasms. Most commonly affects women.

Cause: Unknown. Possible precipitating factors include infection, polymyositis, antigen-antibody reaction in persons receiving chemotherapy as treatment for cancer.

Symptoms and Signs: Many and varied. Swelling, induration, weakness, and inelasticity of muscles; intermittent fever; sore throat; malaise; anorexia; incontinence; diplopia; addisonian discoloration and skin changes, including redness, eruptions, scaling; enlarged spleen; cutaneous lesions overlying the joints of the hands.
Diagnostic Procedures Usually Ordered: Blood chemistry, hemoglobin, sedimentation rate, x-ray.
Treatment: If a tumor is present, treatment of that condition; otherwise, treatment is supportive and symptomatic.
Complications: Heart or respiratory failure.
Course: Chronic and progressive. Prognosis is guarded. Recovery rate, approximately 50 percent.

DIABETES INSIPIDUS

Condition: An uncommon disease characterized by excessive thirst (polydipsia) and the passage of large quantities of urine (polyuria) of low specific gravity.
Cause: A congenital or acquired lesion in the area of the brain that controls the water balance of the body. Deficient secretion (by the posterior pituitary gland) of the antidiuretic hormone (vasopressin), which normally acts on the tubules of the kidneys to control the quantity and concentration of urine excreted, is responsible for the primary symptoms.
Symptoms and Signs: Primary signs are excessive thirst and excessive secretion of pale, very dilute urine. Also, dryness of the skin and mucous membranes of the mouth, constipation, dehydration.
Diagnostic Procedure Usually Ordered: Urinalysis.
Treatment: Vasopressin, the antidiuretic hormone.
Complications: Any of the symptoms listed above may be aggravated by trauma or intercurrent infection.
Course: Chronic. Outcome depends on the cause of the disease and effectiveness of the treatment.

DIABETES MELLITUS

Condition: An absolute or relative failure of certain cells of the pancreas (beta cells of the islands of Langerhans) to secrete sufficient insulin to effect proper metabolism of carbohydrates.
Cause: Often unknown. Contributing factors include heredity, obesity, hormonal imbalance, improper metabolization of iron, pressure

of pancreatic calculi or of a tumor, ingestion of excessive amounts of such concentrated carbohydrates as sugar.

Symptoms and Signs: Numerous and varied. Primary symptoms: weakness; backache; loss of weight; excessive appetite and thirst; cyanosis, especially of the feet; cold, dry, and perhaps yellowish skin (xanthochromia); sometimes, yellowish spots or plaques on the eyelids (xanthelasma).

Diagnostic Procedures Usually Ordered: Urinalysis, blood chemistry analysis, glucose tolerance test.

Treatment: Institution of a dietary regimen to decrease intake of carbohydrates, especially sugar; administration of insulin by hypodermic or, in mild cases (particularly in the elderly), an oral hypoglycemic agent. All other treatment is palliative, supportive, or for the rather numerous and often serious complications that arise in the course of the disease. No known cure.

Complications: Arteriosclerosis, retinitis, cataracts, predisposition to infection, cutaneous lesions (especially of the lower extremities where they sometimes progress to ulceration and even gangrene), acidosis, coma. Insulin shock may occur when a person is receiving insulin therapy.

Course: Chronic and lifelong. Diabetes can usually be controlled with a carefully regulated dietary and medical regimen. Life expectancy has greatly increased since the discovery of insulin.

Prevention: Avoidance of obesity, especially when there is a family history of diabetes; medical advice to diabetic individuals that children of marriages between diabetics are very likely to have the disease.

ERYTHEMA NODOSUM

Condition: An acute, inflammatory skin disease characterized by the appearance of tender red nodules occurring bilaterally in successive patches over a period of several weeks.

Cause: May be unknown. May be a complication of a bacterial, fungal, or viral infection, or a result of drug toxicity. Sometimes associated with scarlet fever, cat scratch fever, roundworm, or sarcoidosis.

Symptoms and Signs: Painful red nodules on the lower legs, fever, malaise, pain in muscles and joints, edema of the skin.

Treatment: Directed to the cause, if known. Antibiotics or corticosteroids may be prescribed. Local treatment not usually effective.

Course: Self-limited, with slow return to normal over a period of weeks.

GOITER (SIMPLE)

Other Name: Colloid goiter.
Condition: Nodular, nontoxic enlargement of the thyroid gland.
Cause: Unknown. Usually thought to be due to insufficient iodine in drinking water or food. Possible precipitating factors include heredity; endocrine influences; certain drugs, including thiouracil, taken by the individual's mother.
Symptoms and Signs: Usually asymptomatic except for visibility of the enlarged gland. When enlargement is severe there may be symptoms produced by pressure on adjoining structures. May be accompanied by hypothyroidism or hyperthyroidism, with symptoms of these conditions.
Diagnostic Procedures Usually Ordered: Basal metabolism rate, radioactive iodine metabolism, cholesterol determination.
Treatment: If treated early, iodine therapy may be effective. Replacement therapy if accompanied by hypothyroidism. Surgery if pressure on adjoining structures warrants it or if accompanied by hyperthyroidism.
Complications: If the goiter becomes very large, the patient will have difficulty in swallowing, dyspnea on exertion, displacement of the trachea, and paralysis of the laryngeal nerve. Rarely, Graves' disease or cancer.
Course: Usually first appears in adolescence, enlarges gradually until middle age, and then gradually subsides. Usually responds favorably to treatment.

HEMOCHROMATOSIS

Common Name: Bronze diabetes.
Condition: A disorder of iron metabolism characterized by the deposit of iron-containing pigment in the tissues, especially the liver and the skin. Occurs most often in men, seldom before the age of 40.
Cause: Unknown. Thought to be a hereditary trait.
Symptoms and Signs: Many, the most common being a gray and/or brown pigmentation of the skin, the gray being due to iron, the brown to melanin. Also, weight loss; general weakness; lassitude;

painful muscles and muscle cramps, especially in the legs; enlargement of the liver.

Diagnostic Procedures Usually Ordered: Blood chemistry, bone marrow examination for hemosiderin.

Treatment: Therapy is directed toward the removal of excess iron, usually by weekly phlebotomy (500 ml), until the hematocrit is normal or shows a mild deficiency of iron.

Complications: Cardiac failure, cirrhosis of the liver.

Course: Most patients respond well to the phlebotomy regimen. Prognosis is guarded.

HEMOSIDEROSIS

Condition: A chronic, progressive disorder characterized by deposition of hemosiderin (an iron-containing pigment) in the tissues, usually the lungs. Similar to hemochromatosis but localized and with a tendency to bleeding, while hemochromatosis is disseminated and there is no tendency to bleeding. Occurs most often in men.

Cause: Unknown.

Symptoms and Signs: The main symptom is recurrent attacks of bleeding (with coughing, dyspnea, and sometimes spitting and vomiting of blood), and consequent anemia. Many other symptoms, including abdominal pain, tachycardia, jaundice, dyspnea, cyanosis, enlarged spleen.

Diagnostic Procedures Usually Ordered: Complete blood count, clotting time, x-ray of the lungs.

Treatment: Symptomatic and palliative. No known cure.

Complication: Heart failure.

Course: Usually fatal.

HYPERPARATHYROIDISM

Condition: An abnormal increase in the activity of the parathyroid glands causing loss of calcium from the bones.

Causes: May be caused by hyperplasia or tumor (benign or malignant); may be a congenital trait.

Symptoms and Signs: Multiple, dependent on the extent of the disease; general muscle weakness is outstanding. Also, anorexia; nausea; constipation; bone pain and skeletal deformities; urinary tract involvement with polyuria, polydipsia, and renal colic.

Diagnostic Procedures Usually Ordered: Blood chemistry, white blood cell count, x-ray.

Treatment: Surgery.
Complications: Spontaneous fractures, renal calculi, uremia, thrombocytopenia, duodenal ulcer, hypercalcemic crisis, parathyroid crisis.
Course: Chronic, with periods of remission and exacerbation.

HYPERTHYROIDISM

Other Name: Graves' disease.
Condition: Excessive production of the thyroid gland hormone; condition is sometimes referred to as exophthalmic goiter, toxic goiter, or thyrotoxicosis. More common in women than men.
Cause: May be unknown. Contributing factors include familial metabolic defect, infectious diseases, psychic or physical trauma, excessive administration of the thyroid hormone, hypothalamic or pituitary dysfunction.
Symptoms and Signs: Usually those associated with increased metabolic rate—restlessness, nervousness, muscular weakness, intolerance to heat, dyspnea, insomnia, palpitation, emotional instability, irritability, increased appetite with loss of weight. Sometimes, anorexia, nausea, vomiting, diarrhea, flushing and sweating, tachycardia, fine tremor of the outstretched hands, protrusion of the eyeballs (exophthalmos).
Diagnostic Procedures Usually Ordered: Blood chemistry, urinalysis (special emphasis on electrolyte and protein waste excretion), radioactive iodine uptake, thyroid scan, thyroid function tests, basal metabolic rate.
Treatment: Depends on age and condition of the patient and severity of the disease. Surgery for younger patients, but not for the elderly. Antithyroid drugs prepare the patient for surgery or irradiation, or for temporary treatment, but are seldom used for long-term therapy. Radioiodine is usually ordered for the older patient. Other treatment is symptomatic.
Complications: Heart failure is the most serious and frequent complication.
Course: Onset usually after age 40, but may occur as early as 30. Persists if untreated, although there may be remissions. Spontaneous recovery may occur, but this is not the rule.

HYPOGLYCEMIA

Condition: A symptom complex resulting from an abnormally low amount of glucose in the blood. May be organic or functional in origin.

Functional Hypoglycemia

Causes: Rapid, excessive intake of carbohydrates which increases the output of insulin; gastric surgery; excitement; ingestion of alcohol; or there may be no apparent cause.
Symptoms and Signs: Same as for the organic form.
Diagnostic Procedures Usually Ordered: Blood sugar levels, glucose tolerance test, examination of urine for glucose.
Treatment: Emergency treatment is the same as for the organic form. Long-term treatment: a diet rich in proteins and low in carbohydrates, with small, frequent feedings; psychotherapy if indicated; such drugs as tranquilizers, sedatives, or anticholinergic preparations.
Complications: Obesity, possibly cerebral ischemia.
Course: Usually self-limited to a few months or years.

Organic Hypoglycemia

Causes: Usually, a tumor of the islands of Langerhans in the pancreas. Also, malabsorption syndrome, hepatic disorders, vomiting, diarrhea, malnutrition, adrenal-cortical-pituitary insufficiency.
Symptoms and Signs: Varied, but hunger, weakness, headache, irritability, anxiety, diplopia, and fainting usually occur.
Diagnostic Procedures Usually Ordered: Blood sugar levels, examination of urine for glucose, electrocardiogram.
Treatment: Emergency treatment the same as for insulin overdosage, namely, administration of sugar in some form. Other treatment is directed at the cause.
Complications: If the condition persists and is not treated, brain damage may occur.
Course: Onset rapid. Usually responds to administration of glucose.

HYPOPITUITARISM

Other Names: Simmonds' disease, pituitary cachexia.
Condition: Failure of the anterior lobe of the pituitary gland to

produce (wholly or in part) its hormones. Occurs chiefly in women.
Causes: Atrophy of the pituitary gland, infection, trauma, hemorrhage.
Symptoms and Signs: Relate primarily to the functioning of the thyroid, the adrenal cortex, and the gonads: anorexia, emaciation, premature aging, loss of body hair, depression of the basal metabolic rate, impotence, mental deterioration.
Diagnostic Procedures Usually Ordered: Basal metabolic rate, radioactive iodine uptake, glucose tolerance test, urinalysis, white blood cell and differential counts.
Treatment: Substitution therapy to provide the needed hormones.
Course: Depends on whether the cause can be and is removed, the amount of damage the gland has sustained, and the adequacy of the therapy.

HYPOTHYROIDISM

Condition: The thyroid gland does not secrete enough thyroid hormone to maintain the proper level of metabolism; the condition produced is often referred to as myxedema.
Causes: Spontaneous hypothyroidism—cause unknown. Thyroid myxedema—may follow surgical removal of part or all of the thyroid gland; thyroiditis, the use of radioiodine.
Symptoms and Signs: Usually, the reverse of those for hyperthyroidism, although some are the same for both conditions. Usually, intolerance to cold; stiffness of the joints; constipation; dyspnea; diminished vigor; hoarseness; slurred speech; puffiness around the eyes; tendency to obesity; cold, dry skin that is yellowish or waxy in appearance; thinning of the eyebrows and hair, which tends to be dry, brittle, and prematurely gray; bradycardia; low body temperature; enlargement of the heart; pleural effusion; ascites; edema of the extremities; mental retardation. Blood pressure may be lowered in younger patients, but is usually elevated in older people.
Diagnostic Procedures Usually Ordered: Circulation time, radioactive iodine uptake, blood chemistry, thyroid scan and function studies, basal metabolic rate.
Treatment: Substitution therapy—thyroid extract or other preparation of the thyroid hormone is usually all that is required. Undesirable symptoms that persist are treated as needed.
Complications: Congestive heart failure, infections, hypothermic coma.
Course: Can be altered by substitution therapy.

LUPUS ERYTHEMATOSUS (SYSTEMIC)

Condition: A chronic disorder characterized by widespread collagen damage to many organs, dermatologic manifestations, and remissions and exacerbations of varying lengths. Occurs more often in women than in men.

Cause: Unknown; appears to be genetic in origin. There are many possible contributing factors, including allergy, drug sensitivity, exposure to sunlight, infections, and stressful situations, including surgery and pregnancy.

Symptoms and Signs: Multiple. *General symptoms* include anorexia, weakness, malaise, loss of weight, low-grade fever, rheumatoid musculoskeletal pain, enlargement of lymph nodes and spleen, abdominal pain, diarrhea, epileptiform seizures. *Blood symptoms*: anemia, thrombocytopenia, leukopenia. *Cardiac symptoms*: myocarditis and pericarditis. *Renal symptoms*: proteinuria, nephritis, pyuria; possibly, renal insufficiency and failure. *Neuropsychiatric symptoms*: nervousness, anxiety, depression. Chief dermatological sign: a symmetrical, erythematous rash, mainly on the face and neck, possibly appearing in a "butterfly distribution" over the bridge of the nose and cheeks; may also extend to other parts of the body and become scaly and pruritic. Other skin signs are urticaria, alopecia, purpura.

Diagnostic Procedures Usually Ordered: Urinalysis, blood evaluation, Coombs test, colloidal gold test, LE cell test, tests for immunological abnormalities, x-ray.

Treatment: Avoidance of sunlight; high-calorie, high-vitamin diet; treatment of intercurrent illnesses; symptomatic treatment during exacerbations and as they arise. Drug therapy includes corticosteroids to suppress the inflammation, salicylates for musculoskeletal pain, iron salts and possibly blood transfusion for anemia, immunosuppressive agents, antibiotics for intercurrent infections.

Complications: Muscle atrophy, necrosis of the bone, glomerulonephritis, hepatitis, heart failure.

Course: Chronic. Prognosis for cure is poor.

PELLAGRA

Condition: A deficiency syndrome affecting mostly the skin, alimentary tract, and nervous system.

Cause: Deficiency of nicotinic acid (part of the vitamin B complex) in the diet; often, a concomitant deficiency of folic acid.

Symptoms and Signs: Varied, but the three "Ds" of pellagra predominate—diarrhea, dermatitis, and dementia. The diarrhea is one of many digestive disturbances; the dermatitis results particularly from exposure to light; the dementia includes emotional instability, disorientation, and depression. The dermatitis appears mostly on the face, neck, arms, hands, and feet; at first it is erythematous and scaly, later vesicles and bullae may develop. Permanent pigmentation of the skin may occur. Other symptoms include anorexia, general debility, spinal pain, stomatitis, glossitis, hypotension, tachycardia.

Diagnostic Procedures Usually Ordered: Blood and bone marrow evaluations.

Treatment: Administration of niacinamide (a compound that acts in the same manner as nicotinic acid but has fewer side effects), a general vitamin preparation that contains all of the vitamin B complex, a well-rounded diet with extra protein, attention to general health.

Course: Response to dietary and vitamin therapy usually favorable. Prognosis in severe and untreated cases is poor.

POLYARTERITIS NODOSA

Condition: A disseminated, necrotizing inflammation of the medium-sized and small arteries and arterioles, resulting in dysfunction of the organ system involved.

Cause: Unknown.

Symptoms and Signs: Many and varied according to the organs affected and the extent of the disease; no one symptom is diagnostic. Fever, skin eruptions, pain in the joints, hypertension, peripheral neuritis, palpable nodules in various parts of the body, various renal disorders.

Diagnostic Procedures Usually Ordered: Urinalysis, complete and differential blood cell count; possibly, muscle biopsy.

Treatment: Symptomatic and supportive; corticosteroids to reduce the inflammation, antibiotics for intercurrent infections.

Complications: Renal decompensation, hypertension, congestive heart failure.

Course: Onset is sudden, prognosis is unpredictable. Unless corticosteroid therapy is effective, the course is apt to be rapidly downhill, with death resulting from one of the three complications listed above.

SCURVY

Condition: A deficiency disorder produced by prolonged insufficient intake of vitamin C.
Cause: Lack of vitamin C in the diet (usually associated with a diet that is poor in fresh fruits and vegetables).
Symptoms and Signs: Multiple. Most commonly, irritation; inflammation and ulceration of the gums; tendency to hemorrhage into the skin, joints, muscles, gums, and subperiosteal areas. Also lassitude, malaise, myalgia, delayed wound healing.
Diagnostic Procedures Usually Ordered: White blood cell, plasma, and urine evaluations for vitamin C; differential count; capillary fragility test.
Treatment: Large amounts of vitamin C, and a well-rounded diet.
Complications: Various infections, particularly tuberculosis; tendency to hemorrhage; defective healing of wounds, fractures, and thermal burns.
Course: Response to treatment usually favorable. When untreated, scurvy can be fatal.

SJÖGREN'S SYNDROME

Other Name: Keratoconjunctivitis sicca.
Condition: A chronic, generalized connective tissue disorder.
Cause: Unknown. Possible contributing factors include allergy, endocrine disorders, autoimmunity, association with rheumatoid arthritis or other collagen disorders.
Symptoms and Signs: Many and varied: lack of tears; photophobia; dryness, stinging, and grittiness of the eyes with stringy mucous discharge; dry nose and mouth with difficulty in swallowing; low-grade fever.
Treatment: No specific treatment known. Therapy is palliative and symptomatic; saline irrigations and artificial tears may help.
Course: Chronic, with frequent remissions and exacerbations.

THYROIDITIS (CHRONIC)

Condition: A progressive, inflammatory disease of the thyroid gland. Most often occurs in women over 60 years of age.
Cause: Unknown.
Symptoms and Signs: Cough, hoarseness, dyspnea, dysphagia, en-

largement and tenderness of the thyroid gland with development of palpable hard nodules, hyperthyroidism.

Diagnostic Procedures Usually Ordered: Biopsy, basal metabolic rate, uptake of protein-bound iodine.

Treatment: Surgery or drug therapy with the administration of thyroxin, depending on the circumstances.

Complications: Abscess formation: hypothyroidism.

Course: Onset is insidious. Prognosis depends on effectiveness of treatment.

VITAMIN DEFICIENCIES

Diseases and disorders caused by insufficient intake of specific vitamins include pernicious anemia (lack of vitamin B_{12}), scurvy (lack of vitamin C), pellagra (lack of nicotinic acid), and rickets (lack of vitamin D and calcium). Unless irreparable tissue damage has occurred, a cure for these disorders can be expected to result from a diet that includes intake of the specific vitamin.

However, a broader vitamin deficiency is not uncommon, especially in older people. The symptoms may not be obvious, but a general subclinical condition exists. Treatment usually consists of administration of multiple vitamin preparations, with or without minerals, of which an almost limitless number is available. The exact preparation the physician chooses will depend on the requirements of the individual person.

RDA stands for recommended daily allowance. The RDA for vitamins is usually listed by percentage on the label of the container. Thus, 100 percent RDA is the amount the Federal Drug Administration has determined is needed by the average healthy adult to retain his good health, but this amount may not be adequate for older persons. Although the RDA has not been established for all vitamins, this does not mean that these vitamins are not essential.

Some vitamin preparations may have the vitamin content listed on the label in milligrams. The milligram labelling gives the vitamin dose by weight, as with any drug. Unit labelling is also used and, in this case, the label states the amount of the vitamin preparation needed to produce a specific result.

Trace minerals are sometimes included in vitamin preparations, and the amounts are listed on the label. Iron is usually included; magnesium, zinc, copper, manganese, and iodine may also be added.

Vitamins A and D are toxic in excessive amounts and should not be taken without medical advice.

WEGENER'S SYNDROME

Other Name: Granulomatosis, Wegener.
Condition: A generalized, granulomatous disorder that is apt to be rather rapidly fatal; affects many organs and structures of the body.
Cause: Unknown. Possible contributing factor: hypersensitivity.
Symptoms and Signs: Symptoms are those of an inflammatory condition; malaise, cough, weight loss, pain in the sinuses, chest pain, rhinorrhea with purulent discharge, nosebleed, hemoptysis. Later symptoms include kidney disorders, uremia, and cardiac insufficiency.
Treatment: No effective treatment known. Corticosteroids may be used; antibiotics for secondary infections.
Course: Onset is insidious. Course generally progressively downhill. Possible survival, 4 to 5 years following appearance of symptoms.

CHAPTER 6

Disorders of the Nervous System

BRAIN DISORDERS

FUNCTIONAL BRAIN DISORDERS

Chronic Brain Syndrome

Other Names: Chronic syndrome, dementia, senile organic brain syndrome.

Condition: A slow deterioration of the higher cortical processes.

Causes: Usually multiple. May include any or several of the following: metabolic disturbances, vascular insufficiency, idiopathic degenerative disease, intoxication, nutritional deficiency, tumor, trauma, congenital anomaly, encephalitis, meningitis.

Symptoms and Signs: Early—lack of initiative, failing memory, feelings of inadequacy, irritability, poor occupational performance, dysarthria. Late—moodiness, poor general comprehension, impairment of judgment, continued memory loss (especially for recent events), aphasia, progressive deterioration of the intellectual functions.

Diagnostic Procedures Usually Ordered: Depend on the suspected cause.

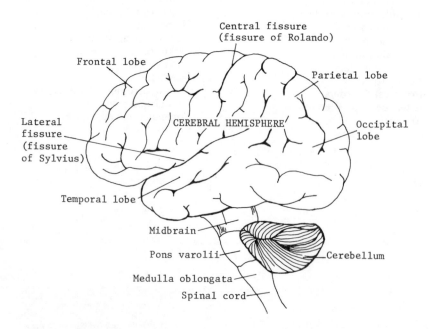

The Brain. Diagram shows the principal divisions, lobes, and fissures.

Treatment: Symptomatic, with psychotropic drugs.
Complications: The etiological condition may progress, or secondary deterioration may occur.
Course: Usually, steadily progressive.

Confusion

Condition: Inability to discriminate in an appropriate manner; occurs in both healthy and sick individuals of any age but more commonly in older persons. Usually transient in healthy individuals, and may be related to unsureness about such factors as the date, time of day, direction, and so on. However, confusion may be a serious disorder, even neuropsychiatric in nature.
Causes: Any of an unlimited number of situations—emotional, mental, or physical. Emotional factors include such strong stress situations as a fire, severe storm, war, bereavement, or separation from a loved one. Confusion based on mental factors has much the same background as that caused by emotional factors. Confusion based on physical factors is rather common and relatively easy to explain; factors include high fever or diseases of the brain, both of which cause the neurons to "misfunction," and delirium results. A single dose (therapeutic or otherwise), excessive doses, or prolonged use of alcohol and/or hallucinogenic drugs, psychotherapeutic drugs, and certain stimulants or depressants can cause confusion in susceptible individuals.

In older persons, confusion may be caused by arteriosclerosis or any condition that interferes with the regular blood supply to the brain. It may be precipitated by such minor factors as change in routine, rearrangement of the furniture, or a visit from someone whom the patient has not seen for a long time. Confusion may also be an early symptom of any toxic condition such as pneumonia, diabetes mellitus, hyper- or hypoglycemia, or hyperthyroidism.
Symptoms and Signs: Failure to recognize relatives or friends of long standing; failure to realize date, time, place, direction, or appropriate behavior; sometimes failure to realize one's own name and address.
Treatment: Usually, removal of the cause is all that is needed. In caring for the elderly, if one anticipates the circumstances that may bring on confusion, informs the patient of what is going to happen, and assures him that there will be someone available to help him adjust to the change, episodes can often be prevented. When confusion occurs, an explanation of what has happened may have to be repeated many times.

Depression

Other Names: Depressive reactions, melancholia.
Condition: An emotional state characterized by a slowing down of physical and mental activities, sometimes to a state of apathy. Easily recognized when severe; may be difficult to recognize when mild. Generally, it is difficult to tell the difference between the many types of depression; most authorities classify it by causative factors or accompanying conditions.
Causes: Sometimes there is no apparent cause. May begin in childhood when parents react unfavorably to the child's hostility and the child learns to suppress feelings, thus programming himself for depression in later life. In adults, may be secondary to such disturbing circumstances as death in the family, divorce or separation from loved ones, or loss of material possessions (for instance, loss of one's home by fire or storm). May be precipitated by chronic or crippling illness; by disease conditions such as cardiac or gastrointestinal disorders, neuromuscular and arthritic conditions, malignancy, tuberculosis, mononucleosis, or viral hepatitis; by stress experienced during the climacteric or following extensive surgery.

Elderly people who live alone and have multiple illnesses and those who take such drugs as the Rauwolfia derivatives or other antihypertensive agents, or methyldopa or similar products, are susceptible. Tranquilizers and sedatives sometimes tend to heighten depression, especially in the elderly.
Symptoms and Signs: Vary from a feeling of uselessness and anxiety to depression so profound that the patient becomes suicidal but does not have enough energy to commit suicide.

Physical signs—fatigue, backache, headache, crying, insomnia, neuromuscular disorders, anorexia, constipation, and gradual reduction in the speed of performing normal activities.

Nonphysical symptoms—feelings of anxiety, helplessness, and worthlessness; tension; retardation; agitation; loss of interest in sex, work, and other activities; emotional unsatisfaction; dependency on others; hypochondria.
Treatment: Depends on many factors, such as age and condition of the patient, cause (if known) and depth of the condition. Removing or treating the cause may be all the treatment needed. When the cause is not known, or when depression persists after the cause has been removed, further treatment may include psychotherapy, possibly the administration of tranquilizers and/or motor stimulants. Severely affected patients may require hospitalization and electro-

convulsive therapy. In chronic cases, when the patient is unable to cope with life problems or is suicidal, hospitalization that provides a sheltered environment is best.

Course: Acute or subacute states respond favorably to adequate therapy, although relapses and recurrences are common. Some patients need intermittent treatment throughout life. Chronic cases need continuous care and treatment.

Paranoia

Condition: A chronic, progressive mental disorder, characterized by systematized delusions, usually of persecution or grandeur.

Cause: Direct cause unknown. Contributing factors are failure to achieve overvalued goals, and various traumatic life experiences.

Symptoms and Signs: *Persecutory type*—patients blame others for their own hostile, aggressive motives; are secretive, vindictive, and depressed; have suicidal tendencies; behave spitefully against others, for whom they feel self-righteous resentment; often write letters to authorities complaining of conspiracies against them.

Litigious type—patients insist on attributing wrongdoing to other people, often the result of legal experiences that were not resolved to their satisfaction; make constant attempts to show the superiority of their own personality.

Erotic type—patients believe they are loved by persons who are wealthy or socially or otherwise prominent and try to gain favors from them by persistent efforts, threats, or even criminal acts.

Treatment: Usually, psychotherapy; tranquilizing drugs or shock therapy may be used.

Course: Depends on the effectiveness of the therapy.

Schizophrenia

Other Names: Schizophrenic reaction; formerly known as dementia praecox.

Condition: A psychosis characterized by severe disruption in normal, logical connection of thoughts and in relationships with others.

Causes: Actual cause unknown. Possible predisposing factors include familial tendency, disruptions in family life (especially those that occur early in life), poor mother-infant relationship, a general inadequate relationship between the child and his parents and siblings, sometimes (especially during adolescence) inability to reach goals that are often unrealistic, or poor school or work accomplishments.

Symptoms and Signs: *Simple schizophrenia*—gradual withdrawal from reality, apathy, inappropriate moods, bizarre behavior, irritability, feelings of rejection, lack of self-respect, undue worry about one's condition, lack of interest in external things, limitation of relationships with others. Delusions and hallucinations are not usually present.

Paranoidal schizophrenia—inadequate personal relationships, coldness, withdrawal, use of sarcasm, scornfulness, defiance, resentment of authority, hallucinations (usually auditory and visual), delusions of persecution but possibly also of grandeur.

Catatonic schizophrenia—disturbances in activity with either stupor or excitement. When excitement is the prevailing mood, motor behavior is unorganized and aggressive; the patient is impulsive, unpredictable, hostile, resentful, and irritable. He sleeps little, refuses food and drink, loses weight, becomes dehydrated and exhausted, and may have hallucinations or delusions of being supernatural and having unlimited power. When stupor is the prevailing state, the patient shows lack of interest and of communication with others, loss of emotionality, muteness, catalepsy, and a mask-like, staring expression.

Hebephrenic schizophrenia—characterized by bizarre mannerisms, silliness, giggling, incoherent speech, fragmented delusions, and affective behavior that is shallow, inadequate, and inappropriate.

Treatment: All types: depends on the degree of regression. In all cases, therapy is prolonged, possibly life-long. For mild cases, psychotherapeutic drugs, psychotherapy, and, if possible, adjustment in the life pattern and home environment. For more severely ill patients, hospitalization is usually indicated; in addition to treatments used for mild cases, hydrotherapy or other physical therapy, possibly electroconvulsive therapy; and, with improvement, work therapy, recreational therapy, or occupational therapy.

Course: Insidious onset, rarely short. Early treatment may result in partial or complete recovery. Prognosis for partial recovery is fairly good, even in patients who have regressed seriously. Most schizophrenic patients need occasional therapy for years, some for life.

Senile Dementia (including Alzheimer's disease)

Other Names: Senile psychosis, diffuse brain atrophy.

Condition: A psychosis associated with old age, characterized by atrophy of the cortex of the brain.

Cause: The process of aging, independent of infection, vascular disorder, metabolic deficiency, or neoplastic disease.

Symptoms and Signs: Varied, but usually include agitation, loss of memory (especially for recent events), narrowing of interests, confabulation, rigidity of views and beliefs, distrust, suspicion. May resemble chronic brain syndrome.

In Alzheimer's disease the symptoms are similar, but may also include greediness, restlessness, shuffling gait, muscular stiffness, awkward movements, epileptiform attacks, abnormal sense perception, aphasia, and sclerosis of the retinal blood vessels.

Diagnostic Procedures Usually Ordered: X-ray, electroencephalogram, brain scan, pneumoencephalogram.

Treatment: Limited to control of agitation with psychotropic drugs.

Course: Symptoms appear slowly and become chronic; mental deterioration is progressive. Prognosis is poor.

Alzheimer's disease is also chronic and progressive; starts much earlier than senile dementia, often in the fifth decade.

ORGANIC BRAIN DISORDERS

Most organic brain disorders occur in the younger person. However, the elderly patient may be subject to any of them. The main difference is that in older individuals these disorders tend to be more severe than in younger persons.

Brain Abscess

Brain abscess may be single or multiple and may be in one location or several. These pyogenic brain conditions are usually the result of an infection elsewhere in the body. Symptoms are those of the original infection plus those due to the effects of the infection on the area of the brain involved. Treatment consists of removal of the cause if known, and, if possible, surgery and/or anti-infective drugs.

Brain Injury

Brain injury may consist of anything from mild concussion to severe, depressed skull fracture. Symptoms vary with the location and severity of the injury. If the condition is mild, prevention of shock may be the only treatment needed. Patients with more severe injury are treated for shock and given needed supportive treatment until surgery can be done.

Brain Tumor

Brain tumor may be benign or malignant (primary or secondary). Symptoms vary with size, type, and location of the tumor. Treatment is palliative, supportive, and symptomatic, and may include surgery or irradiation.

CONVULSIVE DISORDERS

The Epilepsies

Condition: Acquired or congenital neurological disorders characterized by convulsive seizures that result from a disturbance in normal brain rhythm.

Causes: Unknown in most cases. Possible causative factors include heredity, trauma such as birth injury, infection, tumor, vascular pathology of the brain.

Symptoms and Signs: *Grand mal epilepsy*—characterized by irregularly occurring convulsions that follow an immediately preceding aura in which the patient may experience an odd sensation of apathy, nausea, dizziness, ringing in the ears, spots before the eyes, tingling sensation in fingers or toes, and some motor phenomena. The patient loses consciousness, falls, and a tonic convulsion occurs, which may be so severe that the opisthotonus position is assumed. Usually, frothing at the mouth, dyspnea, stertorous breathing or temporary periods of apnea and cyanosis; sometimes, tongue-biting, loss of bladder control, and bruising from the fall. As the seizure abates, the patient breathes in gasps, his muscles are flaccid, and tendon reflexes are absent; consciousness gradually returns, followed by a deep sleep that lasts for hours. Upon awakening, amnesia for the convulsive episode is common.

Status epilepticus—a severe form of grand mal epilepsy; the interval between seizures is very slight or even absent, thus creating an emergency situation that requires energetic treatment.

Jacksonian epilepsy (focal epilepsy)—characterized by irregularly occurring focal or limited convulsions that begin with tingling of fingers or toes, numbness, paresthesia, and muscular twitching, and progress to include one side of the body, rarely the entire body. Consciousness is usually retained unless the convulsion becomes complete.

Petit mal epilepsy (pykno-epilepsy, minor epilepsy)—characterized by short periods of amnesia, myoclonic jerks, cessation of activity. No convulsion, aura, or coma. During episodes, the patient has a staring, vacant expression, may move his eyes or head rhythmically, and occasionally loses bladder control. Two types are recognized: (1) the astatic type, in which there is loss of body control; and (2) the myoclonic or kinetic type, in which the patient may fall, but has no convulsion.

    Psychomotor seizures (epilepsia procursiva, temporal lobe epilepsy, psychomotor convulsion, psychomotor equivalent)—term used to describe convulsive disorders that do not fit into the three main categories of epilepsy. During seizures, any or all of the following symptoms may be noted: pallor, automatism, incoherent speech, turning of the head and eyes, lip smacking, patterned movements (apparently purposeful), twisting and writhing movements, perceptual illusions (sight, smell, taste), hallucinations, partial unconsciousness, postseizure amnesia for the episode.

Diagnostic Procedure Usually Ordered: Electroencephalogram.

Treatment: All forms: drug therapy with anticonvulsants, sedatives, diuretics, and tranquilizers; the exact drug and dosage are highly individualized. During an episode, the only treatment is to prevent the patient from injury insofar as this is possible. Patients need to be encouraged to do all they can but to avoid occupations involving personal danger. Some are helped by psychotherapy, especially those of highly emotional temperament. Status epilepticus is a medical emergency best treated in a hospital; drugs may be administered intravenously.

Complications: Status epilepticus is the most serious complication; mental deterioration, emotional changes, and behavioral disturbances may occur.

Course: Chronic, but not life-threatening (except for status epilepticus). Usually can be wholly controlled, or at least enough to allow the patient to lead a fairly normal life.

NEUROLOGICAL DISORDERS

ARTERIOSCLEROSIS (CEREBRAL)

Condition: Reduction in cerebral function due to impairment of the blood supply to the brain.

Causes: Degeneration of the lining of the arteries and/or atheromatous degeneration secondary to hypertension, endarteritis, or thromboangiitis obliterans.

Symptoms and Signs: Early: headache, dizziness, impairment of vision. Later: progressive loss of intellectual capacity, loss of memory, confabulation, reminiscence, vague delusions, paranoid tendencies, depression; possibly, epileptiform attacks, senile tremor, aphasia, agnosia, apraxia, paraplegia, retinal atheroma.

Diagnostic Procedures Usually Ordered: X-ray, angiogram, brain scan.

Treatment: Symptomatic, with the use of psychotropic drugs.

Complications: Profound dementia.

Course: Chronic and progressive, with discouraging outlook.

ARTERITIS (CRANIAL)

Other Names: Left, right, or bilateral arteritis; temporal arteritis; giant cell arteritis.

Condition: Inflammation of the cranial (temporal) arteries.

Cause: Unknown.

Symptoms and Signs: *Prodromal stage*—anorexia, weakness, sweating, malaise. *Later stages*—severe headache, often unilateral, nocturnal, and intractable; pain in the face, teeth, jaws, and scalp; weight loss; photophobia; amblyopia; diplopia; oculomotor paralysis; ptosis of the eyelids; papilledema; confusion; delirium; polyneuropathy with joint movement. The temporal arteries are prominent and the overlying skin is edematous, reddened, and painful.

Diagnostic Procedures Usually Ordered: Complete blood count, sedimentation rate.

Treatment: Steroid therapy (cortisone derivatives) has been successful in preventing such complications as blindness.

Complications: Cerebral ischemia, blindness.

Course: Usually, the acute condition clears in about two to three months, but decreased visual acuity often persists.

BELL'S PALSY

Other Name: Facial paralysis.

Condition: Paralysis of the muscles on one side of the face.

Cause: A lesion in the facial nerve. Often the cause of the lesion is unknown, but it may be due to infection, trauma, exposure to chilling, or pressure of a tumor on the nerve.

Symptoms and Signs: Pain behind the ears or eyes; facial numbness and heaviness; excessive tearing; drooling; unilateral weakness, spasms, and paralysis of facial muscles; characteristic distortion of the face with one corner of the mouth sagging; patient cannot close the mouth; the forehead is unfurrowed; the palpebral fissure is widened.

Treatment: Avoidance of exposure and chilling, and keeping the face warm; cortisone taken orally may help in emergency situations; decompression of the facial nerve may be required. Other treatment: symptomatic and palliative; sometimes, plastic surgery.

Complication: Rarely permanent paralysis.

Course: Sudden onset. Recovery is usually complete in from two to eight weeks in younger persons, up to two years in older persons. Some patients do not regain full functioning of the involved muscles. Recurrences on the same or opposite side are not unusual.

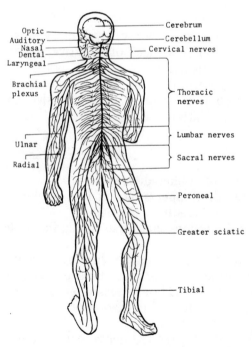

Optic
Auditory
Nasal
Dental
Laryngeal

Brachial
plexus

Ulnar

Radial

Cerebrum
Cerebellum
Cervical nerves

Thoracic
nerves

Lumbar nerves

Sacral nerves

Peroneal

Greater sciatic

Tibial

The Nervous System

CHOLESTEATOMA

Condition: A rare epithelial tissue tumor containing fatlike material; occurs in the ears, eye sockets, pericranium, and on cranial nerve.
Cause: A defect in embryonic development.
Symptoms and Signs: Depend on location and size of the tumors. Facial palsy, pain in the face, deafness, exophthalmos, hemiplegia, convulsions.
Treatment: Surgery when feasible. Otherwise, treatment is symptomatic.

CHOREA

Chronic Progressive Chorea

Other Names: Huntington's chorea, hereditary chorea.
Condition: A degenerative neurological disorder that usually starts in the third or fourth decade of life.
Cause: Hereditary.
Symptoms and Signs: Restlessness; quick, jerky, involuntary movements; disturbances in speech; moodiness; lack of initiative; loss of memory; shuffling gait; mental deterioration.
Treatment: Palliative, with psychotropic drugs. No known cure.
Course: Onset is insidious. Course is chronic and progressive; patients often live from 10 to 15 years after onset.

Senile Chorea

Other Names: Chronic progressive nonhereditary chorea.
Condition: A form of chorea that appears late in life; similar to chronic, progressive chorea but not hereditary in origin.
Cause: Usually, cerebral vascular lesions that occur in middle or old age.
Symptoms and Signs: Unilateral, purposeless, involuntary muscular movements that are rapid, irregular, and jerky; restlessness; lack of initiative; obstinacy; shuffling gait; normal or increased reflexes; usually, a gradual loss of memory but no mental deterioration.
Treatment: Psychotropic drugs as needed.
Complications: Progressive disability; rarely, mental deterioration.
Course: Fairly rapid onset in middle or old age; disability is progressive.

HEADACHE

Headache, one of man's most common ills, may be a symptom, a syndrome, or a disease, according to the circumstances.

Condition: Slight, moderate, or severe pain in any or all parts of the head; may be steady or paroxysmal. Common forms are histamine cephalalgia, tension headache, and migraine syndrome.

Causes: Unlimited. A few representative causes include any cerebral disorder that causes increased intracranial pressure; trauma, especially to the neck, face, or shoulders; hypertension; cranial arteritis; sinusitis; dental disorders; eye diseases; fever; various infectious diseases; loss of fluid by spinal puncture; emotional stress; muscular or psychological tension.

Symptoms and Signs: Nausea, vomiting, dizziness, photophobia, "spots before the eyes" and other visual disturbances, pain. It is important for those who care for patients with headache to note the location and intensity of the pain, the time of onset, whether it is an isolated occurrence or paroxysmal, and the time the pain occurs in relation to eating, sleeping, and other activities of living.

Histamine Cephalalgia

Other Name: Horton's cephalalgia.

Condition: Severe unilateral pain in the head; of sudden onset, often during sleep.

Cause: Dilatation of the anterior and middle cerebral arteries. Predisposing causes are unknown. Excess histamine has not been proven to be the cause, hence the name is incorrect.

Symptoms and Signs: Sudden onset of pain on one side of the head, often occurring during sleep; pain in the eye, temple, face, and neck, and flushing of the face on the affected side; nasal discharge and lacrimation; hypotension; distension and tenderness of the temporal vessels on the affected side.

Treatment: Prevention: methysergide maleate (Sansert) may prevent the episodes. During attacks usually none is needed. For prolonged attacks, which are relatively rare, analgesics may be needed.

Diagnostic Procedures Usually Ordered: Histamine test; examination of cerebrospinal fluid.

Course: Attacks are usually of short duration.

Migraine Syndrome

Other Names: Vascular headache, hemicrania.
Condition: Periodic, paroxysmal attacks of severe headache, usually unilateral but sometimes progressing to involve the entire head; characterized by remissions and exacerbations. More common in women than men; often begins in adolescence.
Causes: Direct cause unknown. Possible causes include familial tendency, endocrine imbalance, abnormal sympathetic innervation of the cranial arteries, hypersensitivity. May be precipitated by emotional or physical stress.
Symptoms and Signs: Prodromal stage: usually, nonpainful sensory disturbances, often visual. Later stages: paroxysmal attacks of pain that start on one side of the head and may remain unilateral or progress to involve the whole head; painful throbbing of cerebral arteries; possibly salivation, tearing, photophobia, visual disturbances, nausea, vomiting, diarrhea, pallor or redness of the face and eyes, scintillating scotomas, excessive perspiration, fever. Attacks may last for a few hours to a few days.
Treatment: Ergotamine tartrate (Gynergen) to abort or prevent attacks; rest for two or more hours after an attack to prevent immediate recurrence.
Complications: Intractable persistent pain, incapacitation.
Course: Chronic, with attacks becoming less frequent and less severe as the patient ages. A lifelong but not life-threatening disorder.

Tension Headache

Other Names: Muscle contraction headache, musculoskeletal headache.
Condition: A common type of headache, which may be severe, moderate, or mild; unilateral, bilateral, or migrating; steady or intermittent; may be precipitated or intensified by exposure to cold.
Causes: Strain on the muscles of the neck, face, or shoulders. Often, no organic cause can be found.
Symptoms and Signs: Contractions or spasms of the muscles of the neck, head or face; tenderness over the affected muscles; often described by patients as bandlike, cramplike, nonpulsating, or as a tightness.
Treatment: Often unsatisfactory. Heat and gentle massage to the affected muscles; analgesics, tranquilizers, or sedatives to relieve the acute attack. Rest, relaxation, and freedom from worry helps most patients; some benefit from psychotherapy.

HERPES ZOSTER

Other Names: Shingles, zona, zoster.
Condition: Inflammation of the spinal nerve ganglia, characterized by pain and crops of reddened vesicles along the distribution path of a sensory nerve.
Cause: A virus.
Symptoms and Signs: Severe pain and eruption along the site of the affected nerve, fever, malaise, chills, headache, paresthesia or hyperesthesia over affected nerve, enlargement and tenderness of regional lymph nodes.
Treatment: Symptomatic, to relieve pain and itching of the vesicles; analgesics may be needed.
Complications: Scarring, severe conjunctivitis with scarring of the cornea if not treated, paralysis of facial nerves, post-herpetic neuralgia.
Course: The vesicular rash becomes cloudy after two to three days, dry and crusted in from five to ten days; it clears in about two weeks. Post-herpetic neuralgia is common and may persist for days, months, or even years, with varying periods of exacerbation and remission.

NEUROGENIC ARTHROPATHY

Common Name: Charcot's joint.
Condition: A form of osteoarthritis characterized by enlargement of the joints, especially the ankle, knee, hip, spine, or hand.
Causes: Trauma; a complication of tabes dorsalis or syringomyelia in which the proprioceptive nerves are destroyed.
Symptoms and Signs: Slightly painful swelling of affected joints; walking may become impossible.
Treatment: Correction of the underlying cause, if possible.
Complication: Dislocation of joint.
Course: Rarely starts in old age but carries over into later years; always chronic but not fatal.

PARKINSONIAN SYNDROME

Other Names: Parkinson's disease; paralysis agitans; shaking palsy.
Condition: A neurological disorder characterized by stiffness of muscles, tremor, and nodding of the head.
Cause: Not usually known. Precipitating cause is loss of functional

activity of some of the basal ganglia, which may be the result of a viral infection, carbon monoxide poisoning, or arteriosclerosis.

Symptoms and Signs: Mild tremor, head nodding, masklike expression, slowness of movements. Later, shuffling gait with festination, stiffening of the muscles, and increase in severity of all symptoms. Mental capacity is not affected.

Treatment: Several drugs are available, but side effects often outweigh benefits; regular exercise; massage. Surgery has been used in some cases.

Course: Chronic and progressive.

POLYNEURITIS

Condition: Inflammation of more than one nerve.

Causes: Mainly, chemical poisons, inadequate diet, excessive use of alcohol, diabetes mellitus, infectious diseases.

Symptoms and Signs: Weakness and muscle cramps, especially of the leg; numbness, tingling, and paresthesia of hands and feet; anesthesia or hyperalgesia.

Treatment: Removal of the cause.

Course: Progressive and chronic.

SCLEROSIS

Amyotrophic Lateral Sclerosis

Condition: A slowly progressive condition characterized by loss of muscle control and use.

Cause: Unknown. May be inflammation of the spinal cord, nutritional deficiencies, or vascular disorders.

Symptoms and Signs: Muscular atrophy; paresis; paralysis, usually of the upper half of the body.

Treatment: None that is curative.

Course: Chronic and progressive. Usually onset is during the fifth or sixth decade of life. Prognosis is poor.

Multiple Sclerosis

Other Name: Disseminated sclerosis.

Condition: A chronic, progressive neurological disorder that usually starts in the second to the fourth decade of life; characterized by hardened patches scattered throughout the brain and spinal cord that interfere with the nerves in those areas.

Cause: Unknown. Possibly, the result of an allergy or a viral infection.

Symptoms and Signs: Disturbances of vision, weakness of extremities, dizziness, headache, myasthenia, paresthesia, incoordination, ataxia, tremor.

Diagnostic Procedures Usually Ordered: Colloidal gold test, ophthalmoscopy; cerebrospinal fluid examination.

Treatment: None that is effective; physical therapy and counseling on the changes required in life patterns are helpful.

Course: Chronic, with the symptoms gradually becoming more incapacitating. Although the disease starts in youth, some patients live as long as 30 years after diagnosis. Periods of remission are usually followed by increase in the severity of the symptoms with eventual complete incapacitation.

TRIGEMINAL NEURALGIA

Other Name: Tic douloureux.

Condition: A chronic, rarely fatal, severe neurological disorder characterized by remissions and exacerbations.

Cause: Unknown. Apparently, irritation of the trigeminal nerve causes the symptoms.

Symptoms and Signs: Brief attacks of severe pain in the face and forehead that may be precipitated by touching certain areas around the nose and mouth, exposure to cold, or eating and drinking.

Treatment: Palliative, with certain drugs that sometimes control the symptoms. If medical treatment fails, surgery may be done, but this is not always effective.

Course: Always chronic, carries over into later years; remissions tend to become shorter as the person ages.

CHAPTER 7

Diseases and Disorders of the Ear and Eye

DISEASES AND DISORDERS OF THE EAR

DEAFNESS

Condition: Partial or complete loss of hearing. Occurs frequently in the elderly. The most common forms involve either a nerve condition or a disturbance in the normal conduction of sound waves through the ear. *Functional deafness* is a form that cannot be traced to an organic lesion. *Mixed hearing loss* is a combination of nerve deafness and conduction deafness (described below).

Causes: *Nerve deafness*—destruction of inner ear structures, the nerve pathways to the brain, or the hearing center in the brain as a result of congenital conditions (trauma, maternal illness, fetal illness, fetal malformation); trauma to the inner ear or the eighth cranial nerve; vascular disorders of the inner ear, the eighth cranial nerve, or the brain centers for hearing; toxic agents (ototoxic drugs, for example); bacterial or viral infections; severe febrile diseases; Meniere's syndrome; tumor of the inner ear or brain; multiple sclerosis; presbycusis; exposure to loud noise.

Conduction deafness—failure of transmission of sound waves from the exterior to the cochlea of the inner ear; may be due to congenital malformation, trauma, otosclerosis.

Diagnostic Procedures Usually Ordered: Audiogram.

Treatment: *Nerve deafness*—no known treatment. *Conduction*

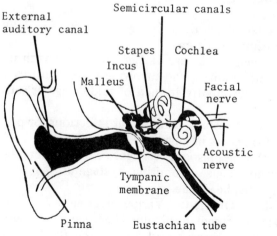

The Ear

deafness—see treatment for otitis externa, otitis media, and otosclerosis.

Complication: Permanence of the condition.

Course: May be reversible during the first months, depending on the cause.

IMPACTED CERUMEN

Condition: An abnormal collection of cerumen (ear wax) in the external ear canal, partially or completely blocking the lumen of the canal.

Causes: A tortuous ear canal, excessive hairs in the canal, dryness or scaling of the skin of the canal.

Symptoms and Signs: In complete occlusion, a sense of fullness and pressure in the ear, deafness on the affected side, possibly tinnitus and a reflex cough.

Treatment: Removal of the cerumen by a physician or someone well qualified to perform the procedure, using an ear curet or irrigation; presoftening may be needed. Serious damage can be done to the ear structures if this procedure is not properly carried out.

Complication: External otitis.

Course: Removal of the cerumen eliminates the symptoms.

MENIERE'S SYNDROME

Other Names: Paroxysmal labyrinthine vertigo, aural vertigo, labyrinthine hydrops, labyrinthine syndrome.

Condition: Repeated attacks of severe vertigo associated with decreased auditory acuity and tinnitus, and involving the structures of the inner ear. Occurs most frequently in men of middle age or early old age.

Causes: Usually unknown. Possibly, trauma, ear infections, or periodic neural dysfunction (as occurs in migraine).

Symptoms and Signs: During episodes—vertigo, tinnitus, decreased hearing acuity, apprehension, nausea, vomiting, nystagmus, diaphoresis. Between attacks—tinnitus, headache.

Diagnostic Procedure Usually Ordered: Various hearing tests.

Treatment: No specific treatment available. Therapeutic measures to control symptoms include measures to reduce the fluid in the labyrinth by means of a salt-free diet and diuretics; controlling the vertigo with antimotion sickness drugs; relieving headache with mild analgesics; and, if indicated, mild tranquilizers to reduce apprehension, a common symptom.

Complication: Deafness.

Course: Chronic, with remissions and exacerbations of varying lengths.

OTITIS

Otitis Externa (acute)

Other Names: Dermatitis of the external ear, topical otitis externa, otomycosis, surfer's ear.

Condition: Inflammation of the external ear, external ear canal, and sometimes the external surface of the tympanic membrane. May be contact dermatitis, seborrhea, or a form of eczema.

Causes: Direct cause—usually a bacterium, less often a fungus. Predisposing factors include the presence of moisture in the ear canal (warm, moist climate, swimming pools, showers); irritation from hearing aids or earrings; scratches due to itching or to attempts to clean the ear.

Symptoms and Signs: Pruritus; pain; tenderness; regional lymphadenopathy; tinnitus; partial or complete deafness; dryness and scaling or a watery to purulent, foul-smelling discharge; fever (may indicate extension of the inflammation); redness and edema of the skin of the external ear and canal). In fungal infections, there may be a velvety membrane, the removal of which lessens the pain.

Treatment: Systemic anti-infective drugs when there is lymphadenopathy and/or fever; mild analgesics for pain. Local treatment consists of keeping the external ear and canal dry and clean and applying medications as indicated by the known or suspected cause.

Complications: Usually none; occasionally the infection spreads to adjacent lymph nodes in the neck.

Course: Tends to be rather persistent and refractory to treatment. Recurrences are common.

Otitis Media (including acute, chronic, and serous forms)

Other Names: Secretory otitis media, chronic otitis media with effusion.

Condition: Inflammation of the middle ear.

Causes: *All forms*—obstruction of the eustachian tube due to sinusitis, nasal or upper respiratory disorders; allergy.

Acute form—rapid descent in the air; lymphoid hyperplasia that blocks the eustachian tube.

Chronic form—often the result of repeated acute infections.

Serous form—may result from inadequate treatment of the acute form.

Symptoms and Signs: *All forms*—sensation of fullness, decrease in auditory acuity, often deafness in the affected ear.

Acute form—earache, feeling of numbness, autophony, an exudate in the middle ear, retracted ear drum.

Chronic form—tinnitus, autophony, and occasionally vertigo; occasionally, perforated ear drum, retracted ear drum.

Serous form—tinnitus, pruritus, tenderness but no pain, bulging ear drum.

Diagnostic Procedures Usually Ordered: Complete and differential blood counts; possibly, culture of excretions with sensitivity testing, audiogram, x-ray.

Treatment: *Acute form*—the usual treatment for infections, including bed rest, analgesics as needed, a suitable anti-infective drug, extra fluids. Additionally, a local or systemic nasal decongestant to aid in opening the eustachian tubes; medicated ear drops; hot or cold local applications; myringotomy when indicated.

Chronic form—improving the functioning of the eustachian tube by treating such underlying conditions as sinusitis, nasal disorders, or other chronic upper respiratory disorders, and following with reconstructive surgery as indicated; applying ear drops and/or drying dusting powder to the external ear canal, particularly when there is drainage from the ear.

Serous form—underlying causes should be removed; nasal decongestants and/or antihistamines to relieve symptoms; possibly, a myringotomy with provision for continued drainage to remove excess fluid.

Complications: Deafness, especially following the serous form. Mastoiditis, labyrinthitis, meningitis may follow the acute form.

Course: *Acute form*—usually short if treatment is effective and no complications arise.

Chronic and serous forms—tend to be chronic; permanent hearing loss is common.

Pseudocholesteatoma

Condition: A relatively uncommon form of chronic otitis media, characterized by the formation of horny, desquamated epithelium and cholestrin crystals in the tympanic cavity; may involve the labyrinth, meninges, brain, or facial nerves.
Cause: Usually, associated with marginal perforation of the tympanic membrane.
Sign: The presence of a hornified mass of epithelial cells as described above.
Treatment: Usually surgery.
Course: Depends on the extent of the deposit and the effectiveness of surgery.

OTOSCLEROSIS

Other Names: Otoporosis, progressive deafness, otitis insidiosa.
Condition: The formation of bony tissue in the capsule of the labyrinth of the ear.
Cause: Unknown; possibly heredity.
Symptoms and Signs: Usually, progressive deafness, tinnitus, and prolonged bone conduction, although the eustachian tube and tympanic membrane remain normal. May also be asymptomatic.
Diagnostic Procedure Usually Ordered: Audiogram; audiometry.
Treatment: Surgery.
Complication: Deafness.
Course: Depends on the effectiveness of the surgery.

PERFORATED TYMPANIC MEMBRANE

Common Name: Ruptured eardrum.
Condition: A break in the tympanic membrane, creating an artificial opening between the external and middle ear. Occurs most often in children, but also may occur in the elderly.
Causes: Usually, infection (otitis media) and trauma.
Symptoms and Signs: Pain, tinnitus; possibly, deafness or bleeding from the laceration.
Diagnostic Procedures Usually Ordered: Otoscopy, audiometry.
Treatment: If healing is not spontaneous, microsurgery may be required.

Complications: Inflammation; deafness in some degree due to interference with conduction; can be partially overcome through use of hearing aids.
Course: Healing is usually spontaneous. Surgical repair may result in improved hearing.

VESTIBULAR NEURONITIS

Other Names: Epidemic vertigo, epidemic neurolabyrinthitis.
Condition: An epidemic disease characterized by vertigo as the principal symptom.
Cause: Unknown; possibly a virus.
Symptoms and Signs: Dizziness, which may be steady or paroxysmal and very disabling; nausea, vomiting, diarrhea, cough, pharyngitis; occasionally, tinnitus and fever.
Diagnostic Procedures Usually Ordered: Complete blood count, with particular attention to atypical mononuclear cells; spinal fluid analysis.
Treatment: Symptomatic.
Complication: Rarely, multiple sclerosis that appears years later.
Course: Usually self-limited, lasting for a day or two. Occasionally there is a residual period of disability that lasts for months or even years and is characterized by fatigue, depression, and varying sensations of disequilibrium.

DISEASES AND DISORDERS OF THE EYE

CATARACT (SENILE) (INCLUDING CORTICAL CATARACT AND NUCLEAR CATARACT)

Condition: Opacity of the crystalline lens of the eye.
Causes: Basic cause—the physiological process of aging. The specific cause of cortical cataract is unknown; gradual sclerosing of the central portion of the lens causes the nuclear type.
Symptoms and Signs: Similar in both forms: progressive blurring of vision, myopia, and polyopia, at first lateral but later bilateral. Stages in the development of cataracts are related to changes in the lens.

   Incipient stage—opaque streaks from the periphery to the center of the lens are seen; the lens remains transparent between the streaks; rarely, dotlike or cloudlike stationary or progressive opacities are seen.

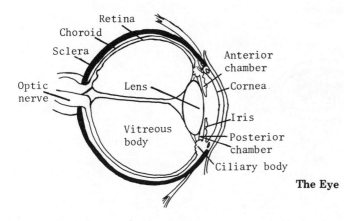

The Eye

Immature stage—the lens is swollen, bluish-white, and shiny, with stellate markings; the depth of the anterior chamber is reduced. With side illumination the shadow of the iris may be seen on the lens.

Mature stage—the lens is gray or amber, and has shrunk in size; opacity is increased. The anterior chamber is of normal depth and the shadow of the iris on the lens during illumination is absent.

Hypermature stage—the lens is homogenous or may present irregular spots; it and the iris are tremulous. The anterior chamber is deepened; the cortex is soft, liquid, milky; the anterior capsule is thickened and opaque.

Diagnostic Procedure Usually Ordered: Ophthalmoscopy.

Treatment: Surgical removal of the cataract (lens) and, in some cases, the substitution of a plastic lens.

Complications: Glaucoma; lens-induced uveitis; if untreated, eventual blindness.

Course: Untreated cataracts progress to blindness. The rate of cure with surgery is high, but sequelae such as retinal hemorrhages may occur.

CONJUNCTIVITIS (CATARRHAL)

Condition: Inflammation of the membrane that covers the eyeball and lines the eyelids.

Causes: Many. In the older person, usually irritation (by dust or smoke, for example) or a decrease in the normal secretion from the lacrimal glands (tears), which results in the eyes not being properly "washed."

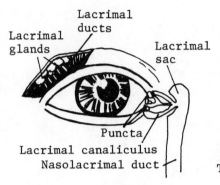

The Lacrimal Apparatus

Symptoms and Signs: Redness of the conjunctiva; smarting, burning, and sometimes itching of the eyelids.
Treatment: Removal of the cause, if possible; eye washes, eye drops, and ointments are used; special preparations containing methylcellulose (artificial tears) may be needed.
Complication: Dissemination to the other eye.
Course: Usually chronic with recurrences.

DEGENERATION OF THE MACULA LUTEA

Condition: Alteration, degeneration, and pigmentation of the macula lutea.
Causes: Often unknown. Contributing factors include familial tendency, congenital anomaly, trauma, ateriosclerosis, old age.
Symptoms and Signs: Bilateral decrease in central vision without loss of peripheral vision; spots are seen on the macula lutea, giving it a "moth-eaten" appearance.
Treatment: No known treatment that is effective.
Complication: Gradual loss of visual acuity.
Course: Chronic and progressive, with eventual total loss of central vision, although peripheral vision is usually unimpaired.

DISORDERS OF THE EYELID

Ectropion

Condition: Outward turning of the upper or lower eyelid; may be unilateral or bilateral. Three types are described—cicatricial, paralytic, and senile.

Causes: Conjunctivitis or blepharitis; spasm or paralysis of the obicularis oculi muscle, especially in the elderly.

Symptoms and Signs: Outward turning of the eyelid; excessive lacrimation; irritation of the lid and conjunctiva; reddening of the conjunctiva; sagging of the lid outward, exposing part of the conjunctiva that is normally covered.

Cicatricial ectropion usually affects both lids bilaterally.

Paralytic ectropion usually affects only the lower lid; may be associated with paralysis of the seventh cranial nerve.

Senile ectropion usually affects the lower lid and simulates the paralytic type.

Treatment: Usually surgery, although the condition may not require treatment.

Complications: Exposure keratitis or corneal ulcers.

Course: Depends upon the type of ectropion and the effectiveness of treatment.

Entropion

Other Name: Blepharelosis.

Condition: Inward turning of the eyelid.

Causes: Many, including scarring following trauma, surgery, burns, or trachoma; prolonged wearing of a bandage; absence or atrophy of the eyeball; spasm of the obicularis oculi muscle; inflammation of the eyelid or conjunctiva; poorly fitted glasses, especially in the elderly.

Symptoms and Signs: Inward turning of the marginal portion of the eyelid, pain, excessive lacrimation, photophobia, congestion, possible opacities of the conjunctiva.

Treatment: Surgery.

Complications: Corneal ulcers; occasionally, trichiasis (ingrowing eyelashes).

Course: Depends on effectiveness of treatment.

DISORDERS OF VISION

Amblyopia

Condition: Dimness of vision due to damage of the optic nerve fibers rather than an organic defect or refractive error.

Causes: Many, some of which may be psychological in origin in addition to those of physiological and pathological origin; toxicity from certain drugs, lead, or alcohol; vitamin A deficiency.
Treatment: Removal of the cause, if possible.
Complication: Permanent impairment of vision in severe types.
Course: Gradual improvement following removal of cause unless damage to the nerve is so severe as to cause permanent impairment.

Astigmatism

Condition: Uneven curvature in some of the refractive components of the eye (cornea, aqueous humor, crystalline lens, vitreous humor), resulting in uneven bending of the light rays; common at all ages.
Causes: Hereditary trait; changes in the cornea resulting from surgery, injury, or inflammation.
Symptoms and Signs: Some objects are seen more clearly than others; a tendency for objects to appear blurred or fuzzy around the edges; headache; pain after using eyes.
Treatment: Correction by specially ground lenses (regular or contact).

Color Blindness

Condition: Inability to distinguish between certain colors; occurs mostly in men—ratio 20:1. Total color blindness (achromatopsia) is rare.
Cause: A sex-inherited trait; may also follow certain diseases, trauma, alcoholic intoxication.
Symptoms and Signs: Most common sign is inability to distinguish between red and green due to lack of ability to identify red (protanopsia) or green (deuteranopsia); rarely, inability to identify blue (tritanopsia), or confusion of blue and yellow.

Hyperopia

Other Names: Hypermetropia; farsightedness.
Condition: The diameter of the eyeball is shorter from front to back than normal, resulting in focusing of light rays behind the retina.
Cause: A hereditary trait.
Symptoms and Signs: To be seen clearly, objects must be held farther from the eyes than is usual; eye strain after close work; headache; possibly, tearing and/or photophobia.

Treatment: Correction with biconvex lenses (regular or contact).

Myopia

Other Name: Nearsightedness.
Condition: The diameter of the eyeball from front to back is longer than normal, resulting in focusing of light rays before they reach the retina.
Causes: A hereditary tendency; possibly nutritional or endocrine disturbance; debility.
Symptoms and Signs: To be seen clearly, objects must be brought closer to the eyes than is usual.
Treatment: Correction with biconcave lenses (regular or contact).

Presbyopia

Condition: Progressive loss of elasticity of the crystalline lens of the eye and lessening of the power of accommodation.
Cause: The aging process.
Symptoms and Signs: Inability to adjust to changes in the distance of objects to be seen; increasing difficulty in seeing near objects clearly without holding them farther and farther from the eyes; ocular pain; tearing.
Treatment: Correction, either with reading glasses with biconvex lenses or bifocal lenses in which part (usually the lower part) is biconvex and part is either regular glass or is ground to correct whatever other eye condition the patient may have.

Strabismus, Esotropia, Exotropia

Condition: The extrinsic muscles of the eyeball do not function properly, resulting in inability to achieve binocular vision or inward turning of one or both eyes toward the nose; rarely seen in the elderly.
Cause: May be hereditary or congenital.
Symptoms and Signs: Reading difficulty; sometimes, diplopia or vertigo.
Treatment: Correction in the elderly can usually be achieved by improving the individual's general health, special muscle training, and possibly surgery, for strabismus; strengthening the muscles or use of corrective lenses for esotropia and exotropia.

GLAUCOMA

Narrow Angle Glaucoma

Other Names: Congestive glaucoma, obstructive glaucoma, closed angle glaucoma.

Condition: Narrowing of the anterior chamber angle with obstructive closure that interferes with the outflow of aqueous fluid and results in increased intraocular pressure. Appears in acute, subacute, and chronic forms.

Causes: Hereditary tendency; possibly, sudden increase in aqueous production; emotional stress. The acute form may be precipitated by the use of a mydriatic.

Symptoms and Signs: *Acute form*—sudden pain in the eye, headache, nausea, and vomiting. Intraocular pressure is increased, eyelids are swollen, the cornea is cloudy, the pupils are fixed and dilated.

Subacute and chronic forms—gradual blurring of vision, slight pain in the eye, headache, hyperopia, patient may see halos around lights. The intraocular pressure is increased, the cornea is cloudy, pupils are dilated and react slowly, the conjunctiva is congested. In the chronic form peripheral vision is lost.

Diagnostic Procedures Usually Ordered: Complete and differential blood counts, tonometry, ophthalmoscopy.

Treatment: *Acute form*—surgery, although miotic drugs may be tried first. *Chronic form*—miotic eye drops.

Complications: Progressive loss of vision with each attack.

Course: If untreated, eventual blindness.

Open Angle Glaucoma

Other Names: Simple, chronic glaucoma; wide angle glaucoma.

Condition: An increased intraocular pressure, resulting in hardening of the eyes, atrophy of the retina and optic disc, and eventual blindness. Accounts for 90 percent of the cases of glaucoma in the elderly.

Cause: Unknown.

Symptoms and Signs: Impairment of vision with partial obliteration of visual form, fields of color, and peripheral vision; diminished adaptation to darkness; colored halos are seen around lights. The anterior chamber is shallow; free granules of pigment are seen in the anterior chamber and on the surface of the cornea; the retinal vessels become obliterated; intraocular pressure is increased; possibly, cup-

ping of the optic disc and excavation of the head of the optic nerve.
Diagnostic Procedures Usually Ordered: Tonometry, ophthalmoscopy.

Treatment: Either surgery or the use of miotic drugs, or both, according to the condition of the eyes and their response to the drug therapy.

Complication: Progressive blindness.

Course: Onset is slow and insidious. Without treatment the condition will progress to blindness.

RETINAL DISORDERS

Detachment of the Retina

Condition: The retina becomes detached, wholly or in part, from the underlying choroid of the eye. May occur at any age but is most common in the elderly.

Causes: Many, including trauma, choroidal exudate or hemorrhage, neoplasms, adhesions due to uveitis or vitreous fibers, cyclitis, chorioretinitis, myopic degeneration, pull on the retina by shrinkage of the vitreous.

Symptoms and Signs: Photophobia, appearance of a dark cloud over the eye.

Diagnostic Procedure Usually Ordered: Ophthalmoscopy.

Detached retina

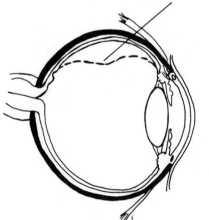

Treatment: Either surgery or the application of the laser beam.
Complications: Secondary glaucoma; possibly, blindness.
Course: Outlook for recovery is good in treated cases. When un-treated, the detachment progresses until the entire retina is detached and opaque, and blindness results.

Retinal Arteriosclerosis

Condition: The walls of the arteries and arterioles of the retina are thickened and hardened, causing a lowering of the blood supply to the retina.
Cause: Usually accompanies general arteriosclerosis, atherosclerosis, or hypertensive disease process.
Symptom: Blurring of vision.
Diagnostic Procedure Usually Ordered: Ophthalmoscopy.
Treatment: Vasodilator drugs are sometimes used, but their effectiveness is questionable.
Complications: Obstruction of the central artery, atrophy of the retina or the optic nerve, thrombosis of the central vein.
Course: Chronic and very slowly progressive.

CHAPTER 8

Diseases and Disorders of the Skin

Diseases of the skin are numerous, varied, and often chronic but, unless malignant, they are seldom life-threatening. For these reasons, many skin disorders that may have started early, even in childhood, are still with the individual in his later years. Few skin disorders start in old age, the most common exception being senile lentigo.

CARCINOMA

Basal Cell Carcinoma (including rodent ulcer)

Condition: Malignant tumor of the skin.
Causes: Unknown. Apparently precipitated by exposure to the rays of the sun, radiation, or arsenic poisoning.
Symptoms and Signs: Small, smooth, macular or papular lesions, with scaling or crusting, that bleed easily, occurring on any part of the body but mostly on the face, scalp, or neck. The lesions of rodent ulcer are slow growing and surrounded with a pearly border.
Diagnostic Procedures Usually Ordered: Biopsy, with cytologic studies.
Treatment: Total excision of the lesions when this is possible.
Complications: Secondary infection, recurrence of the lesions tending toward deeper penetration. Metastasis rarely occurs.
Course: Prognosis is good if the lesions are treated early. Course is progressive when the condition is untreated. Rodent ulcer may destroy a part of the face and prove fatal.

Bowen's Disease

Other Name: Epidermoid interdermal carcinoma.
Condition: A precursor to basal cell carcinoma.
Cause: Unknown.
Symptoms and Signs: A firm, sharply defined, scaling and crusting tumor, single but more often multiple, appearing most frequently on the trunk.
Treatment: Surgical excision.

Epidermoid Skin Carcinoma

Condition: A malignant tumor of the skin.
Cause: Unknown. Possible precipitating factors: chronic irritation,

pipe smoking, leukoplakia, exposure to carcinogens such as tar and arsenic, osteomyelitis.

Symptoms and Signs: Skin lesions that bleed easily, may be warty, nodulated, or ulcerated, may or may not be exudative; occurring chiefly on the nasal mucosa, tongue, exposed areas, or genitalia.

Diagnostic Procedures Usually Ordered: Biopsy, with cytologic studies.

Treatment: Surgical excision, if possible.

Complications: Metastasis to bones, viscera, lymph nodes.

Course: Good possibility of cure if treated early.

Malignant Melanoma

Other Name: Melanocarcinoma of the skin.

Condition: A highly malignant tumor of the skin, occurring usually in white persons.

Cause: Unknown. Possible precipitating factors include an inherited tendency, constant irritation of a pigmented nevus (mole), surgical excision of a nevus.

Symptoms and Signs: Slowly developing skin lesions varying in color—white, tan, pink-rose, brown, black, and usually flat with irregular margins. Course: Depends on the depth of the lesion. Curable only when confined to the primary lesion.

Diagnostic Procedure Usually Ordered: Biopsy, with cytologic studies.

Treatment: Surgical excision if treated early; otherwise supportive and palliative, including chemotherapy to delay recurrences.

Complication: Metastasis.

Course: The survival rate for superficial type is about 70 percent; for the invasive type, about 10 percent; when metastasis has occurred, the usual survival time is 1½ to 3 years.

Sebaceous Gland Carcinoma

Condition: A rare malignant tumor of the sebaceous glands.

Cause: Unknown.

Treatment: Surgical excision.

HERPES SIMPLEX

Common Names: Cold sores; fever blisters.

Condition: The appearance of multiple vesicles (blisters) usually on the lips, but may extend to other tissues.

Causes: The herpes simplex virus. Predisposing or contributing factors include sunburn, abrasions, fatigue, the common cold, extremes of temperature (exposure to cold wind, for example), emotional disturbances.

Symptoms and Signs: Vesicles appear on a reddened, circumscribed area of skin or mucous membrane, usually on the lips or nostrils but also on other parts of the face, the conjunctiva, and the genitalia; pruritus; pain; malaise. The virus may also attack the viscera or the central nervous system.

Diagnostic Procedures Usually Ordered: Complete blood count; analysis of the vesicular fluid; when the nervous system is involved, a spinal tap to obtain cerebrospinal fluid for analysis.

Treatment: No specific treatment. Local application of ointments, creams, or liquid preparations; mild analgesics as needed for pain.

Complications: Infection of the viscera by the herpes simplex virus; encephalitis in susceptible persons.

Course: Self-limited when uncomplicated, lasting from 3 to 14 days. Recurrences are common.

KERATOSIS

Seborrheic Keratosis

Other Name: Acanthotic nevus.

Condition: A form of dermatosis characterized by the appearance of small, sharply marginated, yellowish or brownish lesions covered by a greasy scale.

Cause: Unknown.

Symptoms and Signs: Pruritus, usually mild; characteristic lesions over the trunk, especially the shoulders, scalp, and face; increased pigmentation; granular desquamation.

Diagnostic Procedure Usually Ordered: Punch biopsy.

Treatment: Total excision of the lesions when possible.

Complication: Infrequently, malignant changes in the skin.

Course: Onset usually in later life. Course is persistent, with the lesions rarely disappearing spontaneously.

Senile Keratosis

Other Names: Senile keratoma.

Condition: Thickening, with the formation of horny growth of the outer layers of skin of elderly individuals.
Causes: Often unknown. Contributing factors include congenital ichthyosis, excessive use of lotions or ointments that cause "peeling" of the skin, exposure to the sun's rays for prolonged periods.
Symptoms and Signs: Harsh, dry skin; gradual drying, thickening, and fissuring of the palms and soles. Exposed skin is more apt to be affected than unexposed skin.
Treatment: Cortisone ointment, cream, or lotion; lanolin lotion and bath oils to soften the skin; avoidance of direct exposure to the sun's rays.
Complication: Epidermoid carcinoma.
Course: Calluses and corns may be aggravated. Particularly difficult to manage when the patient has peripheral vascular disease or diabetes mellitus.

LENTIGO (SENILE)

Common Name: Senile freckles.
Condition: Irregular hyperpigmentation of the skin, occurring in older people; usually first seen after age 50.
Cause: The physiological process of aging.
Symptoms and Signs: Small, irregular, circumscribed, brownish, macular patches appearing usually on exposed skin and increasing in number, size, and depth of color as the person ages.
Treatment: Usually none is required.

PEDICULOSIS

Pediculosis Capitis

Condition and Cause: Infestation of the hair of the head with head lice (*Pediculosis capitis*).
Symptoms and Signs: Pruritus; excoriation, and scaling of the scalp; dermatitis; breaks in the skin of the neck and behind the ears; secondary infection from scratching; enlargement of the regional lymph nodes. The nits (ova) can be seen on the hairs. Sometimes the facial hair, including eyebrows, eyelashes, and beard, is also infested.
Diagnostic Procedure Usually Ordered: Microscopic examination of the insect for identification.
Treatment: Many are available, the most common being the use of

gamma benzene hexachloride (Kwell). Usual procedure: shampoo the hair with Kwell and follow with a vinegar rinse that helps to remove the nits.

Complications: Conjunctivitis and corneal ulcers in addition to those listed under Symptoms and Signs.

Course: Usually one treatment is effective; if not, repeat in one week.

Pediculosis Corporis

Condition and Cause: Infestation of the body by the body louse (*Pediculosis humanus corporis*).

Symptoms and Signs: Pruritus, excoriation, and crusting of the skin from scratching; red, elevated papules; in cases of long duration, brownish pigmentation. The lice and nits (ova) are usually seen on the clothing, rarely on the skin.

Diagnostic Procedure Usually Ordered: Microscopic examination of the insect for identification.

Treatment: Same as for scabies. All clothing must be thoroughly washed or dry cleaned after the treatment, as the insects may be found in the seams of clothing.

Course: Depends entirely on the effectiveness of the treatment.

PSORIASIS

Other Names: Willan's lepra; psora; the itch.

Condition: A noninflammatory disease of the skin which may appear at any age except childhood; often first appears during adolescence. A pustular variety is characterized by reddened macules and pustules, often on the thumb and instep.

Causes: Unknown. Contributing factors in the pustular variety are infection, irritation, malnutrition, history of psoriasis.

Symptoms and Signs: Eruption, starting as a single patch, usually on the scalp in the occipital region, spreading as single or multiple papules that appear at hair follicles or sweat pores, possibly with plaque formation, affecting the skin of the knees, elbows, and lumbosacral regions especially, but may appear on skin of any part of the body. Removal of the crusts (silver-gray scales) causes minute bleeding points. Lesions heal without scarring.

Diagnostic Procedure Usually Ordered: "Scotch tape" test for bleeding points.

Treatment: Largely symptomatic; exposure to sunlight; various lotions and ointments, including cortisone ointment. For the pustular variety, treatment is symptomatic.
Complications: Psoriatic arthritis, erythroderma, unfavorable reaction to physical or chemical trauma.
Course: Chronic, with remissions and exacerbations; usually more severe in winter than summer, when it may disappear completely. Does not appear to affect the patient's general health. The pustular variety is resistant to treatment and recurrences are common.

SCABIES

Other Name: Sarcoptic itch.
Condition: A contagious skin disease, characterized by intense itching.
Cause: Infestation of the skin by the itch mite (*Sarcoptes scabiei*).
Symptoms and Signs: Severe nocturnal itching (pruritus) between the fingers and toes, in the folds of the axillae, around the nipples, the intergluteal regions, the umbilicus, and the intercrural areas; excoriations and erythematous patches around the burrows made by the mites; sleeplessness due to itching.
Diagnostic Procedure Usually Ordered: Microscopic examination of skin scrapings.
Treatment: The best of many current therapies is the use of gamma benzene hexachloride (Kwell). A thin layer of the drug is applied after the skin is thoroughly dried following a hot bath using soap liberally. After 24 hours, the ointment is washed off, the person dons clean clothing, and the clothing he has worn during the treatment is washed or dry cleaned.
Complications: Secondary infection from scratching, urticaria, adenitis, pustular eruption, contagious impetigo.
Course: Usually controlled by one treatment as outlined above.

ULCERS

Decubitus Ulcers

Common Names: Pressure sores, bedsores.
Condition: The breakdown of skin, particularly over bony prominences, with the formation of ulcers.
Causes: Decrease in circulation to the area involved. Contributing

factors: any condition that prevents normal movement of the body, long confinement in bed, debilitating diseases, malnutrition.

Symptoms and Signs: Early, erythema; later, blistering and denudation.

Treatment: If ulcer is deep, debridement. Otherwise, various ointments, application of gold leaf, dry heat, prevention of secondary infection.

Prevention: Frequent turning of the patient; good skin care; measures to reduce pressure over bony prominences.

Complications: Infection, gangrene.

Course: The condition is rapidly irreversible unless treated vigorously.

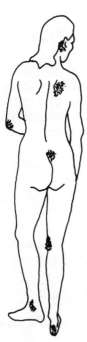

The seven areas where decubitus ulcers (bedsores) are likely to develop.

Varicose Ulcers

Other Name: Stasis ulcers.

Condition: Ulcers on the extremities, associated with varicose veins.

Causes: Chronic insufficiency of venous circulation, often precipitated by trauma.

Symptoms and Signs: Weeping, odorous sore (ulcer), pruritus, pain, warmth of the extremity, tenderness along the course of a vein or veins.

Treatment: Elevation of the extremity to relieve pain; removal of all necrotic tissue and application of a preparation that will encourage granulation, such as granulated sugar, 10 percent Merthiolate, or Congo red; keeping the lesions as dry as possible; preventing secondary infection.

Complications: Muscular contractions, secondary infection, scarring, gangrene.

Course: Depends on effectiveness of the treatment.

CHAPTER 9

Diseases and Disorders of the Genitourinary System

DISEASES AND DISORDERS OF THE URINARY SYSTEM

CYSTITIS (ACUTE)

Other Names: Acute exudative cystitis, acute hemorrhagic cystitis.
Condition: Acute inflammation of the urinary bladder.
Cause: A bacterium such as *Escherichia coli, Streptococcus, Gonococcus,* or *Proteus.* Predisposing factors include such diseases as tuberculosis, moniliasis, syphilis, diabetes mellitus; neoplasms; infections of adjacent organs; chemical irritation.
Symptoms and Signs: Frequency, urgency, and pain and burning on voiding; suprapubic pain; possibly, hematuria.
Diagnostic Procedures Usually Ordered: Urinalysis, urine culture, cystoscopy, x-ray.
Treatment: Administration of proper antibiotic after identification of causative organism, with continued administration until all symptoms have ceased. Other treatment is symptomatic.
Complications: Chronic cystitis, leukoplakia, extension of the infection to the renal area.
Course: Depends on effectiveness of the treatment. Untreated cases usually result in pyelitis or pyelonephrosis.

CYSTITIS (CHRONIC)

Condition: Chronic inflammation of the mucosa of the urinary bladder.

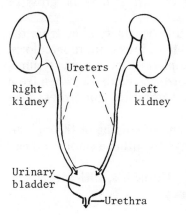

Ureters

Right kidney

Left kidney

Urinary bladder

—Urethra

The Urinary System

Causes: Obstructive lesions, surgical procedures, chronic infectious diseases, radiation, urinary retention.

Symptoms and Signs: Frequency, urgency, and pain on voiding; perineal and/or abdominal pain; drops of red urine following voiding.

Diagnostic Procedure Usually Ordered: Urinalysis, cystoscopy, urine culture, sensitivity tests.

Treatment: Same as for acute cystitis.

Complications: Hemorrhage, systemic infection.

Course: Depends upon severity of the infection, effectiveness of the treatment, and whether complications are present.

GLOMERULONEPHRITIS (CHRONIC)

Condition: Chronic inflammation of the kidneys.

Cause: Usually an acute infection, particularly acute nephritis.

Symptoms and Signs: Headache, weakness, nocturia, weight loss.

Diagnostic Procedures Usually Ordered: Kidney function tests, various blood tests.

Treatment: Maintenance of "good health"; otherwise, treatment is supportive and symptomatic, may include use of the artificial kidney in extreme kidney impairment or a kidney transplant.

Complications: Renal hypertension, circulatory failure.

Course: Survival for 10 to 30 years is common.

HEMATURIA

Condition: The presence of blood in the urine; may be gross or occult. A symptom, not a disease entity.

Causes: Bleeding in some part of the urinary tract; when from the upper part of the urinary tract may be due to infection, tuberculosis, glomerulonephritis, pyelonephritis, neoplasm, infarction, trauma, polycystic renal disease, calculi, or hemorrhagic diathesis; when from the lower part may be due to cystitis, prostatitis, gonorrhea, neoplasm, or calculi.

Sign: Blood in the urine, either at the end of voiding or throughout the entire voiding; small amounts may give the urine a smoky appearance.

Diagnostic Procedure Usually Ordered: Urinalysis, with special emphasis on sediment, color, and translucency.

Treatment: Directed against the cause.

Course: Depends on the cause.

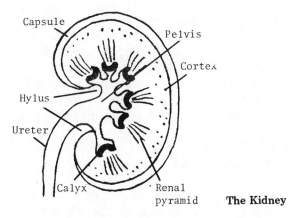

The Kidney

INCONTINENCE OF URINE

Condition: Functional failure of the urethral sphincter, permitting urine to escape from the bladder involuntarily. A symptom, not a disease entity.

Causes: Many, including urinary infections, chronic nephritis, cerebrovascular accident, senile psychosis, loss of nerve control of the sphincter muscle. In women, cystocele or uterine prolapse may cause incontinence; in men, incontinence may be due to prostatitis or other prostatic disorder.

Signs: Involuntary loss of urine, with or without the knowledge of the person; this tendency increases with advancing age. May be a sign of retention with overflow (see retention of urine).

Treatment: The underlying cause is treated or removed, if known. The person should be kept ambulatory, if possible, taken to the bathroom or given a urinal at regular intervals, given psychological encouragement, and not be given any fluids after 6 p.m. if there is nocturnal incontinence.

Complication: Irritation of the genitalia or skin, which may result in decubitus ulcers.

KIDNEY FAILURE (CHRONIC)

Other Names: Chronic renal failure, chronic renal insufficiency (resulting in azotemia or uremia).

Condition: The kidneys fail to remove certain waste products from the blood, resulting in a buildup of these waste products in the bloodstream.

Causes: Many, including chronic glomerulonephritis or pyelonephritis, renal or multiple myeloma, benign or malignant nephrosclerosis, hemoglobinuria, diabetes mellitus, nephrosis, hypertension, hydronephrosis, acute heart failure, myocardial infarction, trauma, fulminating infections, calculi, tumors, or any obstructive nephropathy.
Symptoms and Signs: *Gastrointestinal symptoms*—anorexia, nausea, vomiting, metallic taste, diarrhea, possibly bleeding from the mucosa later.

Urinary symptoms—possibly polyuria in the early stages; later, oliguria that progresses to absolute or relative anuria or nocturia.

General symptoms—headache, fatigue, weakness, thirst, malaise, lumbar pain; in later stages there may also be muscle twitching and/or cramps, late convulsions, generalized edema, anemia, nasal bleeding, "uremic frost" on the skin, petechiae, uremic breath, pruritus, dyspnea, hyperpnea, confusion.
Diagnostic Procedures Usually Ordered: Complete blood count with serum analysis; urinalysis, chest x-ray, kidney biopsy; possibly, spinal fluid analysis.
Treatment: Not usually very effective unless such underlying causes as dehydration or diabetes mellitus can be eliminated or treated. General health measures, including physical and mental activity; low-protein diet with restriction of salt (except in cases of hypotension); correction of electrolyte imbalances; treatment of symptoms as they occur. The anemia which sometimes occurs does not respond to usual antianemic therapy; transfusion may be required if the hemoglobin falls below 8. Kidney transplant is not usually advised for the older patient. Renal dialysis may be used.
Complications: Hypertension, hypertensive encephalopathy, fibrinous pericarditis, congestive heart failure, convulsions, coma.
Course: Depends on age and condition of the patient and whether the underlying cause or precipitating factor can be removed. Onset is insidious, course is usually progressively downhill.

PYELONEPHRITIS (ACUTE)

Other Name: Acute pyelitis.
Condition: An acute bacterial invasion of the pelves of the kidneys and at least part of the parenchyma. More common in men than in women.
Causes: Almost any bacterium (enterococcus or staphylococcus, for example), but chiefly the gram-negative enteric bacilli. Often follows instrumental invasion of the bladder.

Symptoms and Signs: Chills, fever, pain and tenderness in the area of the kidneys, anorexia, nausea, vomiting, dysuria, frequency, urgency.

Diagnostic Procedures Usually Ordered: Urinalysis, urine culture, sensitivity tests, x-ray.

Treatment: Appropriate anti-infective drugs as soon as causative agent is determined; continued for two weeks, when the urine culture is repeated.

Complications: Continuance of the condition with repeated attacks of chronic pyelonephritis and destruction of the parenchyma of the kidney. Hypertension may be a sequel.

Course: Recovery from a single attack is usual. Repeated episodes may lead to renal failure.

PYELONEPHRITIS (CHRONIC)

Condition: Pathological deterioration of the kidneys resulting from repeated episodes of bacterial invasion of the renal pelves and adjacent parenchyma.

Causes: Any one of a number of bacteria, but chiefly the gram-negative enteric bacilli.

Symptoms and Signs: Anorexia, weight loss, fatigue, chills, sweating, fever, tenderness at the costovertebral angle, splenomegaly.

Diagnostic Procedures Usually Ordered: Urinalysis, intravenous or retrograde pyelogram.

Treatment: Similar to that for acute pyelonephritis.

Complications: Hypertension, uremia, renal failure, intercurrent infection.

Course: Insidious onset and course. Outcome depends upon the number and severity of the episodes and whether complications develop.

RENAL CALCULI

Other Names: Nephrolithiasis, urolithiasis.

Common Name: Kidney stones.

Condition: The formation and presence of calculi (stones) in any part of the urinary tract, chiefly in the kidney.

Causes: Unknown. Factors contributing to formation of stones include gout; infections, especially chronic infections; excessive intake

of milk, alkali, or vitamin D; hyperparathyroidism; sarcoid; disorders
of the bone that cause hypercalciuria.

Symptoms and Signs: May be asymptomatic unless the stones
cause obstruction. With obstruction, urinary output is decreased, and
the passage of the stone through the ureter or urethra produces
severe pain.

Diagnostic Procedures Usually Ordered: Urinalysis, x-ray, SMA 18
serum for calculi.

Treatment: In some cases, none is required. Analgesics to relieve
pain and vasodilators may be used. Surgical removal of stones is
sometimes required.

Complications: Depend on the size, number, and location of the
calculi. Hydronephrosis, pyonephrosis, bilateral obstruction with resulting anuria and uremia.

Course: Depends on effectiveness of the treatment and the number
and severity of the complications.

RETENTION OF URINE

Condition: Urine is held in the bladder longer than is usual or
necessary; complete retention occurs rarely. A symptom, not a disease entity.

Causes: Obstruction, compression of the neck of the bladder, nerve
injury, poliomyelitis, general anesthetics; possibly, psychogenic factors. In women, retention may follow gynecological operations of
labor and delivery; in men, it may be due to enlargement of the
prostate gland.

Symptoms and Signs: Usually, a desire to void but inability to do
so; distention of the bladder; dribbling (retention with overflow).

Diagnostic Procedure Usually Ordered: Urinalysis with special emphasis on microscopic examination of sediment.

Treatment: Bed patients are helped to the bathroom or commode
for voiding; hot baths; warm Sitz baths. Catheterization and retention catheters are avoided when possible, since they may cause infection of the bladder.

Complications: Infection; muscular atrophy of the bladder resulting from overdistention.

GENITAL DISEASES AND DISORDERS
OF THE MALE

EPIDIDYMITIS (ACUTE)

Condition: Inflammation of the prostate and seminal vesicle.
Causes: Infectious disease, including gonorrhea or tuberculosis, possibly syphilis or mumps.
Symptoms and Signs: Chills, fever, scrotal and inguinal pain and tenderness.
Treatment: Local heat, support of the scrotum, appropriate anti-infective drugs.
Complications: Sterility (if bilateral involvement), chronic epididymitis.
Course: Usual outcome is favorable. Recurrence may necessitate surgery.

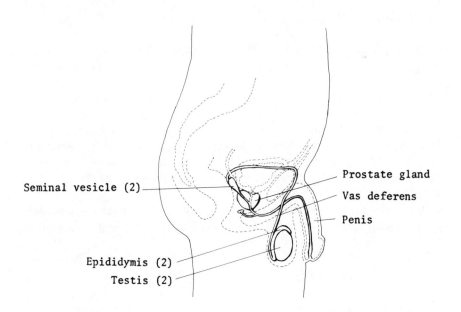

The Reproductive System—Male

HYDROCELE (INCLUDING HYDROCELE OF SPERMATIC CORD OR TESTIS)

Condition: The accumulation of fluid in the tunica vaginalis.
Cause: Often unknown; among many are hernia, infection, and trauma.
Symptoms and Signs: May be asymptomatic. Possibly, scrotal swelling; dragging sensation; interference with walking.
Treatment: Surgery if the condition warrants it. Often no treatment is needed.
Complications: Atrophy of testis; chronic hydrocele.

HYPERTROPHY OF THE PROSTATE (BENIGN)

Other Names: Nodular hyperplasia of the prostate, prostatism.
Condition: Nonmalignant enlargement of the prostate gland with overgrowth of tissue cells. Most common in men over 60 years of age.
Causes: Usually unknown. Possibly a hormonal imbalance with absolute or relative hypersecretion of estrin, calculi, congenital anomalies.
Symptoms and Signs: Sometimes asymptomatic. Frequency, nocturia, dysuria, hematuria, retention with overflow or acute retention resulting from obstruction are common. Sometimes, perineal pain.
Diagnostic Procedures Usually Ordered: Urinalysis with special emphasis on microscopic examination of sediment, intravenous pyleogram, palpation of the prostate gland by rectal examination.
Treatment: Usually surgery.
Complications: Infections of the urinary tract (cystitis, pyelonephrosis, nephritis), obstruction with partial or complete retention of urine.
Course: Surgical results depend on condition of the patient and whether infection develops following surgery.

MALIGNANT TUMORS

Carcinoma of the Prostate

Other Name: Adenocarcinoma of the prostate.

Condition: A malignant tumor of the prostate gland. Occurs most frequently in elderly men.

Causes: Direct cause unknown. Administration of androgens to a patient with prostatic cancer may cause acceleration of the cancerous process.

Symptoms and Signs: The same as those for benign hypertrophy of the prostate plus those of cancer, including frequency, urgency, dysuria, incontinence, retention with overflow, small stream of urine, suprapubic fullness, perineal and bone pain, loss of weight, nausea, tenderness in the renal area. The gland becomes hard, irregular, and nodular.

Diagnostic Procedures Usually Ordered: Urinalysis, blood chemistry, biopsy, x-ray, palpation of the gland by rectal examination.

Treatment: Usually surgery; estrogen may be used.

Complications: Urinary obstruction; uremia; metastasis to regional lymph nodes and pelvic bones, spine, or head of the femur; perineal invasion.

Course: Depends on whether surgery is done before metastasis occurs.

Carcinoma of the Testis

Condition: A malignant tumor of the testis; appears in several forms which vary in severity.

Cause: Unknown.

Symptoms and Signs: Chills, fever, scrotal pain and tenderness.

Treatment: Surgery; irradiation and/or chemotherapy.

Complications: Invasion of surrounding tissues and organs, metastasis to lung and/or liver.

Course: Outlook is unfavorable; possible survival time, 5 years.

GYNECOLOGICAL DISEASES AND DISORDERS

BENIGN TUMORS

Adenofibroma of the Breast

Condition: A benign tumor of the breast.

Cause: Unknown.

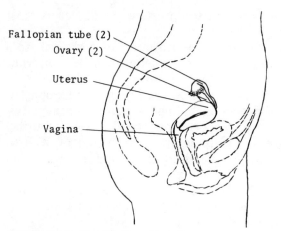

The Reproductive System—Female

Symptoms and Signs: Firm, painless, freely movable nodule that decreases in size with age. May be asymptomatic.

Diagnostic Procedures Usually Ordered: Mammography, biopsy.

Treatment: If asymptomatic, usually no treatment is required. Some physicians advise surgical removal of even small adenofibromas as a preventive measure.

Course: May undergo malignant changes.

Cystic Breast Disease

Other Names: Chronic cystic mastitis, fibrocystic disease.

Condition: A benign cystic tumor of the breast; may be single or multiple, unilateral or bilateral. Often first found on routine physical examination.

Symptoms and Signs: May be asymptomatic; possible discomfort if cysts are numerous and large.

Treatment: If asymptomatic, no treatment is required. If cysts cause discomfort, surgery may be required.

Course: Possibility of malignant change, 1 to 6 percent.

Leiomyoma of the Uterus

Other Name: Uterine fibroids.

Condition: A benign tumor of the body of the uterus composed of muscle and fibrous tissue; may be single or multiple.

Causes: Unknown, possibly hyperestrinism.
Symptoms and Signs: May be asymptomatic and only discovered on routine physical examination. Possibly, lower abdominal fullness; pain; a palpable mass.
Treatment: Surgery, especially for the postmenopausal patient with uterine bleeding.

Ovarian Cystadenoma

Condition: A nonmalignant, slow-growing tumor of the ovary, frequently bilateral; often first discovered during routine physical examination.
Cause: Thought to arise from pathological changes in the surface epithelium of the ovary.
Symptoms and Signs: Early, abdominal pain. Later, abdominal distention, postmenopausal bleeding, large fixed or movable pelvic mass, ascites.
Treatment: Surgery.

CYSTOCELE

Other Name: Cystovaginal hernia.
Condition: Herniation of the posterior part of the urinary bladder into the vaginal vault.
Causes: Usually, obstetrical trauma; possibly, congenital weakness of the pubocervical fascia.
Symptoms and Signs: A sensation of fullness and looseness of the vagina that is increased as a result of long standing, exercise, or fatigue; a palpable, soft, bulging mass in the anterior vaginal wall; stress incontinence if the herniation is extensive.
Diagnostic Procedure Usually Ordered: Urinalysis utilizing a catheterized specimen.
Treatment: Preferred method, surgical repair. Use of a pessary may provide temporary relief until surgery can be performed or for patients whose age and condition precludes surgery. Treatments for bladder infections are the same as for cystitis.
Complications: Chronic cystitis; possibly, pyelitis, hydroureter, hydronephrosis.
Course: Depends upon effectiveness of the treatment.

MALIGNANT TUMORS

Carcinoma of the Breast

Condition: A malignant tumor that originates in breast tissue.

Cause: Unknown. Hyperestrinism may be a causative factor.

Symptoms and Signs: A palpable, hard, fixed or movable mass in the breast; usually painless, especially in the early stages. Possibly, retraction of the nipple, lymphedema, hardening and fixation of lymph nodes in the axillary or supraclavicular region. When untreated, ulceration through the skin with bloody discharge usually occurs.

Diagnostic Procedures Usually Ordered: Blood chemistry, mammography, biopsy.

Treatment: Major treatment is surgery. Other therapies include irradiation, bilateral ovariectomy, administration of testosterone.

Complications: Local or distant metastases.

Course: Survival rate is good (about 75 percent) if regional lymph nodes were not involved before surgery was performed; otherwise, the five-year survival rate is about 30 percent.

Carcinoma of the Uterine Cervix

Other Names: Epidermoid carcinoma of the cervix, adenocarcinoma of the cervix.

Condition: A malignant tumor that originates in the cervix of the uterus. Rarely occurs in women who have not borne children.

Causes: Direct cause, unknown. Possible contributing factors include chronic irritation, estrinism, herpes, penile smegma, leukoplakia of the cervix.

Symptoms and Signs: Early, symptoms may be absent and the cervix may appear normal on examination. Possible signs include leukorrhea and intermenstrual, postmenopausal, or postcoital bleeding. Later, pain in the lumbar region and thighs, weight loss, urinary symptoms, a fixed pelvic mass, erosion or ulceration of the cervix.

Diagnostic Procedures Usually Ordered: Biopsy, colposcopy, x-ray, Papanicolaou smear.

Treatment: Surgery or irradiation, depending on the stage at which the condition is discovered.

Complications: Metastasis to the pelvic bones or regional lymph nodes; invasion into the colon, vagina, or uterine body; formation of fistulas into the colon or bladder.

Course: Insidious, with gradual onset. Survival rate is excellent when the tumor is treated early and vigorously; poor if the tumor has invaded other organs or metastasized.

Prevention: Gynecological examination yearly (or better, every six months), including Papanicolaou smear (test), which will reveal malignant changes in cells early enough for surgical removal of an incipient tumor to be curative in practically all cases.

PROLAPSE OF THE UTERUS

Other Name: Uterus descendus.

Condition: Downward displacement of the uterus, usually described according to degree: *first degree prolapse—*the cervix is located between its normal position and the vaginal opening; *second degree prolapse—*the cervix may be seen at the vaginal opening; *third degree prolapse—*the uterus is outside the vulva; when it is completely outside, the condition is called *procidentia.*

Causes: Often due to stretching and tearing of tissues during childbirth. May be due to congenital anomaly or inherent weakness of the perineum.

Symptoms and Signs: Usually, low backache, a sensation of pressure in the pelvis, dysuria, frequency, leukorrhea. In third degree prolapse, the cervix is often ulcerated, edematous and hemorrhagic; cystocele, rectocele, ureterocele, enterocele, and laceration of the perineum may occur.

Treatment: Depends upon the degree of prolapse and condition of the patient: surgery (hysterectomy); surgical repair if the degree of displacement is slight; a pessary may be used temporarily to hold the uterus in place.

Complications: Depend on severity of the displacement and are related primarily to the urinary system: cystitis, pyelitis, obstruction of the urinary tract with resulting hydronephrosis.

Course: Descent of the uterus is slow and progressive, with prolapse occurring years after the patient has given birth.

RECTOCELE

Other Name: Rectovaginal hernia.

Condition: Herniation of a portion of the rectum into the posterior vaginal wall; usually first noticed several years after the last childbirth.

Causes: Usually, obstetrical trauma. Possibly, congenital weakness of the structures involved.

Symptoms and Signs: Often not diagnostic. Constipation, sensation of fullness in the pelvis, difficulty in emptying the lower bowel, a bulging mass in the upper posterior vaginal wall.

Diagnostic Procedure Usually Ordered: X-ray.

Treatment: Usually, surgical repair. Weight reduction if indicated, correction of constipation.

Course: Surgery usually affords a cure.

CHAPTER 10

Chemical Disorders

ALCOHOLISM (ACUTE AND CHRONIC)

Condition: In the older person, alcoholism is more apt to be chronic than acute, that is, alcohol is used daily with an ever-increasing amount of intake.

Causes: Many precipitating factors are involved, both physical and psychological; possibly, heredity.

Symptoms and Signs: Frequently, vitamin B deficiency due to inadequate food intake; irreversible brain damage if the condition is of long standing; gastritis caused by irritation of the gastric mucosa.

Treatment: *Acute episodes*—vitamin B complex; a well-balanced diet; tranquilizers; balancing of electrolytes, if indicated, by intravenous or oral administration of electrolytes along with glucose. Between episodes the patient is referred to Alcoholics Anonymous or other agency, is provided with counseling, and may be given disulfiram (Antabuse) to help him stop drinking.

Chronic alcoholism—same as for the acute form, except that it is important to try to improve the individual's physical and mental health, which are generally under par, making him subject to infections (especially of the respiratory tract).

Complications: *Chronic alcoholism*: gastritis; portal cirrhosis; degeneration of the optic nerve.

Acute alcoholism: Impairment in cardiovascular and gastrointestinal functions; pneumonia; convulsions (chiefly in epileptics).

Course: *Acute alcoholism*: Episodes repeated at varying intervals; occasionally, death due to respiratory depression.

AMPHETAMINE TOXICITY

Condition and Cause: A state of habituation from continued use of a drug in the amphetamine group that had originally been prescribed or used for cerebral stimulation or for appetite depression in a weight-reduction program. (Their use is now restricted almost entirely to the treatment of narcolepsy and behavioral problems in hyperkinetic children.) Tolerance for the drug results in its use in ever-increasing amounts.

Symptoms and Signs: Apprehension, excitement, restlessness, insomnia.

Treatment: Gradual withdrawal of the drug; possibly, mild sedatives or tranquilizers during withdrawal; measures to improve the individual's general health and habits; psychotherapy.

Complications: Paranoid delusions.
Course: Improvement on withdrawal of the drug.

BARBITURATE TOXICITY

Acute Barbiturate Toxicity

Condition and Cause: Poisoning due to an accidental or intentional overdose of a barbiturate drug.
Symptoms and Signs: Vary according to the amount of drug ingested. Possibly only drowsiness, disorientation, ataxic gait. With larger amounts, stupor and coma; unless treated, death may ensue.
Treatment: Gastric lavage, drugs to improve respiration, digitalis if the cardiac condition warrants it. Other treatment is symptomatic and supportive.
Complications and Course: Central nervous system depression, respiratory arrest, pulmonary edema if coma is prolonged. Barbiturate drugs taken along with alcohol may have a fatal result.

Barbiturate Addiction

Condition and Cause: Dependency on the continued use of a barbiturate drug originally prescribed or used for such conditions as apprehension, anxiety, or a prepsychotic state, after the condition no longer requires its use.
Symptoms and Signs: Vary with the amount of drug taken and length of time it has been used. Insomnia, requiring increasing dosage to overcome it; confusion; inability to continue working at one's normal occupation; social malfunctioning; depression that resembles chronic alcoholism.
   Withdrawal symptoms include anxiety, tremors, ataxia, convulsions; abrupt withdrawal can be fatal.
Treatment: Slow withdrawal of the drug; possibly the substitution of another sedative or tranquilizer during withdrawal; measures to improve general physical and psychological health.
Complications: Dysarthria, nystagmus, mental dullness, frank psychosis. Since the habitué uses the drug to overcome his inability to face the problems of life, his outlook needs to be changed before any real cure can be achieved.
Course: Highly variable because of the many factors involved in habituation.

Chronic alcoholism: Chronic, relapsing, and progressive; loss of control of intake of alcohol with increasing impairment of physical and mental health.

CARBON MONOXIDE TOXICITY

Condition: The replacement of oxygen in the hemoglobin of the red blood cells with carboxyhemoglobin.
Cause: Inhalation of excessive amounts of carbon monoxide in gas from a stove or heater, or in exhaust fumes from an automobile, in an area that is inadequately ventilated. Smog in the atmosphere can lead to chronic carbon monoxide poisoning.
Symptoms and Signs: Headache, breathlessness, nausea, vomiting, confusion, fainting, respiratory arrest if treatment is not instituted early.
Diagnostic Procedures Usually Ordered: Blood tests for carbon monoxide; complete urinalysis; electrocardiogram; electroencephalogram.
Treatment: Remove the person from the area, administer oxygen, institute artificial respiration if indicated.
Complications and Course: If exposure to the gas has been relatively brief, recovery is usually rapid and complete. If exposure has lasted for more than a short period, central nervous system depression, liver complications, and acute renal failure may ensue. Chronic anemia may follow long exposure to smog.

DIGITALIS TOXICITY

Condition and Cause: Digitalis is excreted very slowly and, unless the dosage is kept low, it tends to accumulate in the body and result in toxicity.
Symptoms and Signs: Early signs include anorexia, nausea, and vomiting; later, diarrhea; still later, various cardiac arrhythmias.
Treatment: Early, discontinuing the drug until the excess can be excreted may be all that is needed. Later, hospitalization may be needed for treatment of cardiac complications.

DIURETIC TOXICITY

Condition and Cause: The chief toxicity from diuretics is caused by electrolyte imbalance. The more commonly used diuretics—the thiazides, and the newer (and stronger) drugs, furosemide (Lasix) and ethacrynic acid (Edecrin)—cause the excretion of potassium, sodium, chlorides, bicarbonates, and water in varying amounts. Excessive excretion of potassium is most apt to cause difficulty, especially when a diuretic is taken over a long period of time in the treatment of hypertension or the edema of chronic cardiac decompensation.

Symptoms and Signs: Moderate hypokalemia may be asymptomatic, but as the level of potassium goes down, fainting is not uncommon and heart block or other adverse symptoms may occur. When digitalis is also being taken, symptoms of digitalis poisoning may occur at the same time.

Treatment: Measures to correct electrolyte imbalance.

Prevention: A diet that is rich in potassium, to prevent hypokalemia (bananas, raisins, citrus fruits, and potatoes contain a considerable amount; all fruits and vegetables contain some); the use of "potassium-sparing" drugs such as spironolactone (Aldactone), triamterene (Dyrenium), potassium chloride in liquid form, usually in fruit juice or water, or potassium in tablet form.

SALICYLATE TOXICITY

Condition and Causes: Poisoning caused by the ingestion of a large amount of a salicylate drug, usually aspirin (acetyl salicylic acid), at one time, or the long-time overuse of aspirin or aspirin-containing drugs. Acute poisoning is usually seen in children who find "baby" aspirin and eat it as candy. Chronic poisoning is usually seen in adults who take aspirin alone or in drugs that are highly advertised for arthritis, headache, and muscular aches and pains, and which contain large amounts of aspirin.

Symptoms and Signs: *Acute poisoning*—heart depression, polyuria, impaired hearing or vision, acidosis, bleeding from gastric or other mucous membranes.

Chronic poisoning—nausea, vomiting, small gastric hemorrhages leading to occult blood in the stools, reactivation of an old or partially healed ulcer, tinnitus, dizziness; possibly, skin rash and petechiae.

Treatment: Intake of the drug is discontinued; elimination of the salicylate is induced by stimulating diuresis and other measures; symptoms are treated as they occur.

APPENDIX **A** | Medical Terminology

The medical profession has been said to have the largest specialized vocabulary of any of the professions or vocations. However, it is one of the easiest to learn, since a great majority of the medical words in everyday medical and paramedical use are formed from a rather small number of word fragments called "word elements." For example, the word "gastroenterostomy" can be broken down into "gastro" meaning stomach, "entero" meaning intestine, and "stomy" meaning a surgical opening. Hence, the word means "a surgical opening between the stomach and intestine."

Sometimes the dissection of a word is complicated slightly by the fact that the final vowel of the prefix may be omitted before a suffix that begins with a vowel. For example, myalgia is separated into "myo" (muscle) and "algia" (pain), with the "o" in "myo" being omitted for ease in pronunciation. Likewise, carditis is dissected into "cardio" (heart) and "itis" (inflammation), with the vowels "i" and "o" being omitted before the suffix "itis."

When one understands the definitions of the various word elements, a needed word may be constructed by using the following process:

1. Define the condition for which the medical term is required. For example, suppose the word needed is one that means "a condition of the blood characterized by an increased sugar content."
2. Select the appropriate suffix; in this case the suffix should mean "condition of the blood," that is, "emia."

3. Choose an appropriate prefix; in this case, "hyper," which means increased.
4. Next choose a word element meaning sugar, in this case, "glyco."
5. Arrange the prefixes in the order of increasing importance; in this instance, sugar is more important than increased, so the order should be: "hyper," then "glyco," followed by the word element "emia"—hyper-glyco-emia.
6. Now drop all the hyphens and, as noted above, omit the vowels before the suffix, which begins with a vowel, and the word becomes "hyperglycemia."

Most of the technical terms used in the medical and allied professions are derived from Greek or Latin. This leads to some confusion, since there are often two prefixes or suffixes that have the same or similar meaning. For example, "-algia" (pain) is derived from the Latin, while "-dynia" (pain) is derived from the Greek. Sometimes these suffixes are used interchangeably, but often one is preferred over the other to express slight difference in meaning.

PREFIXES AND SUFFIXES COMMONLY USED IN MEDICAL TERMINOLOGY

a-; ab-	away from; deficient; without
a-; an-; ar-	absent; deficient
adeno-	relating to a gland
aero-	air
-algi; -algia	pain
amb-	both; on both sides
ante-	before
ano-	anus
anti-	against
apo-	opposed
arthro-	joint or joints
-atrics	specialty
aut-; auto-	self
bi-; bis-	twice; double
bio-	life; living
brachio-	arm
brady-	slow
card-; cardio-	heart

-cele	tumor; cyst; hernia
cephal-	referring to the head
cervico-	neck
cholecysto-	gallbladder
chrom-	color
-cide	causing death
circum-	around
contra-	against
cranio-	skull
cyst-; cysto-	bag; bladder
dactyl-	finger
de-	from; not
dent-	relating to teeth
derma-; dermato-	skin
dia-	through; between; across; apart
diplo-	double
dis-	negative; apart; absence of
-dynia	pain
dys-	difficult; bad
ec-; ecto-	referring to the outside
-ectomy	a cutting out
ef-; es-; ex-	out; outside
-emesis	vomiting
-emia	blood
endo-; ento-	within
entero-	intestine
epi-	upon; above
-esthesia	sensation
eu-	well
extra-	beyond; on the outside
fore-	in front of
-fuge	to drive out
galact-; galacto-	milk
gaster-; gastro-	stomach
-gene; -genesis; -genic	origin; production; formation
glosso-	relating to the tongue
glyco-	sugar
-gog; -gogue	to make flow
-gram	a tracing or mark
-graphy	a writing or record
gyn-	pertaining to women
hem-; hemato-; hemo-	relating to blood

hemi-	half
hepa-; hepar-; hepato-	liver
hetero-	other; indicates dissimilarity
holo-	all
homo-; homeo-	same; similar
hydra-; hydro-	relating to water
hyper-	over; above; increased
hypo-	under; decreased
-iasis	condition
-iatrist	specialist
-iatry	field of medicine
idio-	peculiar to an organ or individual
ileo-	ileum
in-	in; not
infra-	beneath
inter-	between
intra-	within
iso-	equal
-itis	inflammation
juxta-	near
kera-	horn; hardness
-kinesis	motion
lact-	milk
laparo-	relating to the loin or abdomen
laryng-; laryngo-	the larynx
latero-	side
leuco-	white
-lith	stone
-logy	study; science
-lysis	dissolution; destruction
macro-	large
mal-	bad; poor; disordered
med-; medi-	middle
mega-	large
melan-; melano-	black
meno-	menstruation
mes-; meso-	middle
meta-	after
-meter	measure
metra-; metro-	uterus
micro-	small
mono-	single

multi-	many
my-; myo-	muscle
myel-; myelo-	marrow
myxo-	mucus
neo-	new
nephr-; nephro-	kidney
neu-; neuro-	nerve
non-	no; not
nucleo-	a nucleus
ob-	against
oculo-	the eye
-oid	resemblance; shape
oligo-	few; scanty
-oma	a tumor
omo-	shoulder
oophoro-	the ovary
ophthalmo-	the eye
orchid-	testicle
ortho-	straight; normal; relating to bones or joints
os-	a mouth; a bone; an opening
-osis	condition; disease
osteo-	referring to bone
-ostomy	to furnish with a mouth or outlet
oto-	the ears
-otomy	a cutting into
pachy-	thick
pan-	entire
para-	along side of; beyond
-path; -pathy	disease; disorder; abnormality
pedi-	pertaining to children
-penia	lack
per-	through
peri-	around
phlebo-	pertaining to veins
-phobia	fear
-phylaxis	protection
-plegia	a stroke
pleura-	the pleura
pneu-; pneuma-; pneumo-	pertaining to lungs or their function
podo-	foot
poly-	many

post-	after
pre-	before
procto-	the colon or rectum
pseudo-	false
psych-; psycho-	the mind
py-; pyo-	pus
-ptosis	a falling or lowering
recto-	rectum
retro-	backward
-rhaphy	a suturing or stitching
rhino-	nose
-rrhea; -rrhage	flow or discharge; hemorrhage
sacro-	sacrum
salpingo-	fallopian tube
sarco-	flesh
sclero-	relating to the sclera; hard
-sclerosis	hardness
-scopy	to see; to look at
semi-	half
soma-	body
stomato-	a mouth
-stomy	to furnish with a mouth or outlet
sub-	under
super-; supra-	above
syn-	together; with
tachy-	fast; rapid
-tension	blood pressure
thera-	treatment
thoraco-	chest
thyro-	thyroid gland
-tomy	cutting
tracheo-	trachea
trans-	across
-trophic	relating to nourishment
uni-	one
-uria	the urine
uro-	urine or urinary organs
vaso-	a blood or lymph vessel
ventro-	the abdomen

COMMON MEDICAL ABBREVIATIONS
AND ACRONYMS

a c	before meals
ad lib	as desired
A/G	albumin-globulin ratio
a m	morning
amt	amount
BE	barium enema
bid	twice a day
BMR	basal metabolic rate
BP; B/P	blood pressure
BRP	bathroom privileges
BUN	blood urea nitrogen
c̄	with
C	Centigrade
cal	calorie
cap	capsule
cath	catheter
cc	cubic centimeter
CHO	carbohydrate
comp	compound
CSF	cerebrospinal fluid
cx	cervix
dc	discontinue
D & C	dilatation and curettage
disch	discharge
Dx	diagnosis
ECG (EKG)	electrocardiogram
EEG	electroencephalogram
EENT	ears, eyes, nose, and throat
elix	elixir
EMG	electromyogram
EST	electroshock therapy
ext	extract
FBS	fasting blood sugar
fl	fluid
fx	fracture
GB	gallbladder
GI	gastrointestinal
gm	gram

gtt	drop
HEENT	head, ears, eyes, nose, and throat
hgb	hemoglobin
H_2O	water
hs	bedtime
Hx	history
I & D	incision and drainage
IM	intramuscular
imp	impression
I & O	intake and output
IV	intravenous
IVP	intravenous pyelogram
kg	kilogram
L	liter
liq	liquid
LP	lumbar puncture
mcg	microgram
mEq	milliequivalent
mg	milligram
ml	milliliter
neg	negative
no	number
non rep	do not repeat or refill a prescription
NPN	nonprotein nitrogen
NPO	nothing by mouth
NSR	normal sinus rhythm
O_2	oxygen
OD	right eye
OR	operating room
OS	left eye
OT	occupational therapy
OU	each eye
p c	after meals
PCV	packed cell volume (hematocrit)
PE	physical examination
p m	afternoon, evening
p o	by mouth
preop	preoperatively
p r n	as needed
Pt	patient
postop	postoperatively
prep	prepare; preparation

q d	every day
q h	every hour
q i d	four times a day
q s	quantity sufficient
R	rectal; right
RBC	red blood cell count
RC	retention catheter
rec	rectum
rep	repeat (refill a prescription)
R_x	prescription; recipe
SC	subcutaneous
Sig	let it be marked (labeled)
SOB	short of breath
sol	solution
spec	specimen
stat	at once
STS	serological test for syphilis
subcu	subcutaneous
surg	surgery
T & A	tonsillectomy and adenectomy
tab	tablet
t i d	three times a day
TPR	temperature, pulse, and respirations
tr	tincture
Tx	treatment
ung	ointment
vit	vitamin
VS	vital signs
WBC	white blood cell count
WC	wheelchair
wt	weight

Weights and Measures Used in Computing Dosages of Medications

Unfortunately, two systems of weights and measures are used in the writing of prescriptions and in medical orders for institutionalized patients, and a third system—the household system—is used in the home care of the sick.

The older system of weights and measures is the apothecaries' system. The metric system, first adopted in France, is rapidly gaining acceptance in the United States and will eventually displace the apothecaries' system entirely. The units in the metric system are based on a decimal system and thus are simpler to use in computing dosages.

Table 1.   Metric and Apothecaries' Weights and Measures: Most Commonly Used Units

Liquid

10 milliliters (ml.) = 1 centiliter (cl.)
100 centiliters (cl.) = 1 liter (L.)
1000 liters (L.) = 1 kiloliter (Kl.)

Weight

10 milligrams (mg.) = 1 centigram (cg.)
100 centigrams (cg.) = 1 gram (Gm.)
1000 grams (Gm.) = 1 kilogram (Kg.) or 1 kilo (K.)

Length

10 millimeters (mm.) = 1 centimeter (cm.)
100 centimeters (cm.) = 1 meter (M.)
1000 meters (M.) = 1 kilometer (Km.)

Liquid

60 minims (𝔪lx) = 1 fluid dram (fl.ℨ i)
8 fluid drams (fl.ℨ viij) = 1 fluid ounce (fl.℥ i)
16 fluid ounces (fl.℥ xvi) = 1 pint (pt. i or O. i)
2 pints (pt. ii or O. ii) = 1 quart (qt. i)
4 quarts (qt. iv) = 1 gallon (cong. i or gal. i)

Weight

60 grains (gr. lx) = 1 dram (ℨi)
8 drams (ℨviij) = 1 ounce (℥i)
12 ounces (℥xii) = 1 pound (lb. i)

Liquid and Weight Conversions

1 minim (𝔪i) = 1 grain (gr. i)
1 fluid dram (fl.ℨi) = 1 dram (ℨi)
1 fluid ounce (fl.℥ i) = 1 ounce (℥i)

Table 2. Conversion Tables for Temperature, Weight, and Length

Temperature				Weight				Length			
°F.	°C.	°C.	°F.	lb.	Kg.	Kg.	lb.	in.	cm.	cm.	in.
0	−17.8	0	32.0	1	.5	1	2.2	1	2.5	1	.4
95	35.0	35.	95.0	2	.9	2	4.4	2	5.1	2	.8
96	35.6	35.5	95.9	4	1.8	3	6.6	4	10.2	3	1.2
97	36.1	36.	96.8	6	2.7	4	8.8	6	15.2	4	1.6
98	36.7	36.5	97.7	8	3.6	5	11.0	8	20.3	5	2.0
99	37.2	37.	98.6	10	4.5	6	13.2	12	30.5	6	2.4
100	37.8	37.5	99.5	20	9.1	8	17.6	18	46	8	3.1
101	38.3	38.	100.4	30	13.6	10	22	24	61	10	3.9
102	38.9	38.5	101.3	40	18.2	20	44	30	76	20	7.9
103	39.4	39.	102.2	50	22.7	30	66	36	91	30	11.8
104	40.0	39.5	103.1	60	27.3	40	88	42	107	40	15.7
105	40.6	40.	104.0	70	31.8	50	110	48	122	50	19.7
106	41.1	40.5	104.9	80	36.4	60	132	54	137	60	23.6
107	41.7	41.	105.8	90	40.9	70	154	60	152	70	27.6
108	42.2	41.5	106.7	100	45.4	80	176	66	168	80	31.5
109	42.8	42.	107.6	150	68.2	90	198	72	183	90	35.4
110	43.3	100	212	200	90.8	100	220	78	198	100	39.4

°F. to °C.: 5/9 (°F. −32)   1 lb. = 0.454 Kg.   1 inch - 2.54 cm.
°C. to °F.: (9/5 x °C.) + 32   1 Kg. = 2.204 lb.   1 cm. = 0.3937 inch

Table 3.   Approximate Dosage Equivalents for Grains, Grams and Milligrams

Grains gr.	Grams Gm.	Milligrams mg.	Grains gr.	Grams Gm.	Milligrams mg.	Grains gr.	Grams Gm.
1/600	.0001	0.1	1/20	.003	3	1½	.100
1/500	.00012	0.12	1/15	.004	4	2	.130
1/400	.00015	0.15	1/12	.005	5	2½	.150
1/300	.0002	0.2	1/10	.006	6	3	.200
1/250	.00025	0.25	1/8	.008	8	4	.250
1/200	.0003	0.3	1/6	.010	10	5	.325
1/150	.0004	0.4	1/4	.015	15	7½	.500
1/120	.0005	0.5	1/3	.020	20	10	.650
1/100	.0006	0.6	3/8	.025	25	15	1
1/80	.0008	0.8	1/2	.032	32	30	2
1/60	.001	1	3/4	.050	50	45	3
1/30	.002	2	1	.065	65	60	4

Table 4.   Approximate Equivalents for Commonly Used Apothecaries' and Metric Units

Apothecaries'	Metric
15 minims (℔xv) or 15 grains (gr. xv)	= 1 milliliter (1 ml.) or 1 gram (1 Gm.)
1 dram (ℨi)	= 4 grams (4 Gm.)
1 ounce (℥i)	= 30 grams (30 Gm.)
1 pint (pt. i or O. i)	= 500 milliliters (500 ml.)
1 quart (qt. i)	= 1000 milliliters (1000 ml.) or 1 liter (1 L.)
1 grain (gr. i)	= 60 milligrams (60 mg.)
$\frac{1}{60}$ grain (gr. $\frac{1}{60}$)	= 1 milligram (1 mg.)
2.3 pounds (lb. 2.3)	= 1 kilogram (1 Kg.) or 1 kilo (1 K.)

Table 5.   Household Equivalents for Apothecaries' and Metric Measures

Household	Apothecaries'	Metric
1 teaspoonful (1 tsp.)	60 drops (gtts.) or 1 dram (ℨi)	4 milliliters (4 ml.)
1 dessertspoonful	2 drams (ℨii)	8 milliliters (8 ml.)
1 tablespoonful (1 tbsp.)	4 drams (ℨiv)	15 or 16 milliliters (15 ml. or 16 ml.)
2 tablespoonfuls (2 tbsp.)	1 ounce (℥i)	30 milliliters (30 ml.)
1 teacupful	6 ounces (℥vi)	180 milliliters (180 ml.)
1 tumblerful	8 ounces (℥viii)	240 milliliters (240 ml.)
1 pint	16 ounces (℥xvi)	500 milliliters (500 ml.)
1 quart	32 ounces (℥xxxii)	1000 milliliters (1000 ml.)

APPENDIX C

Evaluation of Activities of Daily Living (Including Chart)

This Chart may be used for *initial* evaluation of the patient's performance of Activities of Daily Living (A.D.L.), and for *follow-up* observation of clinical progress or retrogression.

The activities which the patient is (or is not) able to perform provide an important index of his functional capacity. However, determination cannot be made simply by eliciting answers from the patient or by simulating motions. Rather, the patient is graded according to observation *during actual performance* of each task. Do not grade activities not so observed.

Grading symbols

G = good (independent, at least fairly efficient)
F = fair (very slow, insecure, tiring)
P = partial (requires supervision or some assistance)
O = zero (not even partial performance possible)

ACTIVITY	INSERT DATE→	1	2	3	4
HYGIENE					
Brush or comb hair					
Brush teeth					
Wash hands					

From *A Guide to Geriatric Rehabilitation* by Herman Kamenetz, M.D., a service manual made available by Armour Pharmaceutical Company. Copyright 1971 by Scicom, Inc., Stamford, Connecticut.

ACTIVITY	INSERT DATE→	1	2	3	4
HYGIENE					
Wash face					
Wash feet					
Turn faucet					
Take shower					
Use handkerchief					
EATING					
Eat with spoon					
Eat with fork					
Use knife					
Butter bread					
Drink (cup, glass)					
WRITING, READING					
Write by hand					
Use typewriter					
Letter into envelope					
Unfold newspaper					
Hold book, turn pages					
LOCOMOTION					
Chair, sitting down					
Chair, getting up					
Room walking					
Stairs up					
Stairs down					
Walk, turn corner					
Get into car					

ACTIVITY	INSERT DATE→	1	2	3	4
DRESSING					
Undershirt, bra					
Shorts, panties					
Shirt, blouse					
Trousers, skirt					
Socks, stockings					
Slip on shoes					
Tie laces					
Jacket, dress					
Zipper, buttons					
MISCELLANEOUS					
Light switch					
Doorknob					
Use drawer					
Dial telephone					
Count coins					
Use scissors					
Use keys					
Move chair					

APPENDIX D

Evaluation of Range of Motion (Including Chart)

Before exercises are instituted for the older person, an evaluation of his abilities should be done. This can be accomplished in several ways, but the two main steps in evaluation involve finding answers to the following sets of questions:

1. What can he do for himself? Can he dress himself, groom himself, feed himself? Can he use the phone? Can he walk up and down stairs? Can he get into a car without help or with minimal assistance? Is he ambulatory? Does he need to use a wheelchair? Is he in bed part time, most of the time, or all the time?
2. Does he have motion in the various joints? How much? If motion in any or several of the joints is impaired, does it appear to be remediable or a permanent loss?

The accompanying charts can be used as a guide for securing information needed to evaluate range of motion of various joints. It is possible for the individual to estimate his own range of motion simply by active movement involving the joints. However, a much more accurate determination of ROM is obtained when passive motion is used by the physician, physical therapist, or nurse.

When it has been determined what the individual can do, exercises can be instituted to maintain this level of musculoskeletal activity and, in many, if not most cases, increase it.

The accompanying evaluation chart can be used as a guide. Specific needs must be met by exercises prescribed by the physician or physical therapist.

This Chart may be used for *initial* evaluation of the patient's joint mobility, and for *follow-up* testing to observe clinical progress or retrogression.

Joint mobility is tested by *passive* execution of motion. Notations on the Chart shall indicate, in degrees of a circle, either the residual capability or the existing limitation. The imprinted degrees of range are approximate norms for individuals of advanced age.

Additional annotations may be made by symbols to indicate muscle tightness **(T)**, weakness **(W)**, spasm **(S)**, or contracture **(C).**

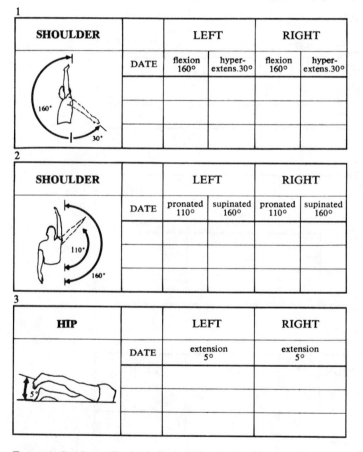

From *A Guide to Geriatric Rehabilitation* by Herman Kamenetz, M.D., a service manual made available by Armour Pharmaceutical Company. Copyright 1971 by Scicom, Inc., Stamford, Connecticut.

4

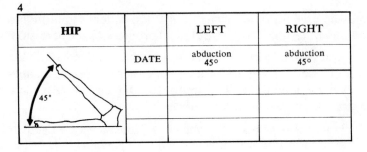

HIP		LEFT	RIGHT
	DATE	abduction 45°	abduction 45°

5

HIP FLEXION		LEFT		RIGHT	
	DATE	straight knee 90°	bent knee 125°	straight knee 90°	bent knee 125°

6

KNEE (flexion)		LEFT	RIGHT
	DATE	flexion 100°	flexion 100°

7

ANKLE FLEXION		LEFT		RIGHT	
	DATE	plantar 40°	dorsal 10°	plantar 40°	dorsal 10°

8

ANKLE		LEFT		RIGHT	
	DATE	inversion 35°	eversion 25°	inversion 35°	eversion 25°

9

GREAT TOE proximal phalange		LEFT		RIGHT	
	DATE	flexion 35°	hyper-extens.80°	flexion 35°	hyper-extens.80°

10

GREAT TOE distal phalange		LEFT	RIGHT
	DATE	flexion 50°	flexion 50°

11

WRIST rotation		LEFT		RIGHT	
	DATE	pronation 90°	supination 90°	pronation 90°	supination 90°

12

WRIST HINGE		LEFT		RIGHT	
	DATE	palmar 80°	dorsal 70°	palmar 80°	dorsal 70°

13

WRIST (radial, ulnar)		LEFT		RIGHT	
	DATE	radial 10°	ulnar 60°	radial 10°	ulnar 60°

14

THUMB proximal phalange		LEFT	RIGHT
	DATE	flexion 70°	flexion 70°

15

THUMB distal phalange		LEFT	RIGHT
	DATE	flexion 90°	flexion 90°

16

FINGER FLEXION proximal phalange		LEFT				RIGHT			
	DATE	Digit 2 90°	3 90°	4 90°	5 90°	2 90°	3 90°	4 90°	5 90°

17

FINGER HYPER-EXTENSION proximal phalange		LEFT				RIGHT			
	DATE	Digit 2 30°	3 30°	4 30°	5 30°	2 30°	3 30°	4 30°	5 30°

18

FINGER FLEXION middle phalange		LEFT				RIGHT			
	DATE	Digit 2 120°	3 120°	4 120°	5 120°	2 120°	3 120°	4 120°	5 120°

19

FINGER FLEXION distal phalange		LEFT				RIGHT			
	DATE	Digit 2 80°	3 80°	4 80°	5 80°	2 80°	3 80°	4 80°	5 80°

APPENDIX E | Exercises For the Elderly

HERMAN L. KAMENETZ, M.D.

Chief, Physical Medicine and Rehabilitation,
State Veterans Hospital, Rocky Hill, Conn.;
Formerly, Asst. Clin. Prof. of Physical Medicine,
Yale University School of Medicine.

EXERCISES FOR THE ELDERLY

The human organism, different from the machine, improves its functions by working. Exercise maintains the flexibility of the joints, improves blood circulation, increases breathing ability, and maintains the strength of muscles necessary to keep the spine in proper position and to maintain the usefulness of all moving parts of the body. Most of all, exercise helps keep the heart in shape.

Age and illness impose some limitations on the normal daily activities, the good 'work out' the body gets even without engaging in special exercises. There are ways to make up for it, to get the necessary 'work out' despite these limitations. The following describes some of these ways, designed to make the elderly *feel less elderly*.

From *Exercises for the Elderly* by Herman L. Kamenetz, M.D., a service manual made available by Armour Pharmaceutical Company. Copyright 1971 by Scicom, Inc., Stamford, Connecticut.

THE GROUND RULES

Exercise and overexertion are two different things. Overexertion is bad for the young and even worse for the elderly. The purpose of the exercise is to *get rid of muscle pain,* not to increase it; to *create relaxation,* not anxiety; to *train the lungs,* not to exhaust them; to *improve circulation,* not to tax the heart. Therefore, remember these ground rules:

• Do the exercises regularly, daily. It's a matter of *building up* your capabilities, not to put them to a test.

• Don't rush. Start slowly, do things at your own pace, *feeling comfortable* doing it. You may allow yourself 15 minutes to an hour to do your bit.

• A little heart pounding and panting after an exercise is normal as long as it doesn't continue for longer than a couple of minutes following the exercise.

• Exercises are best done two times each day: on arising in the morning and before going to sleep for the night. The morning exercises can begin while still in bed (lying position exercises) and they go along well with 'morning stretching.' They take the stiffness out of the joints and the sleepiness out of the muscles. The evening exercises will put a little fatigue into the muscles which enhances relaxation and helps set the stage for a restful sleep.

• As much as you're physically able, try any and all of the exercises described below, then choose the ones you prefer (either for fun or because they help you most) and do them every day.

Here's where the fun begins. However, in your first session do the following exercises (and possibly not all of them) only once. With more practice you can increase the number of repetitions.

Lying Down Exercises

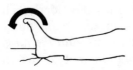

Toe Moving. Curl (flex) all toes as far as you can and then straighten them out as far as you can.

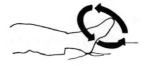

Foot Circling. Make a circle with your foot keeping your heel on the bed, (later off the bed), first in one direction, then in the other. Exercise with each foot separately, later with both feet at the same time.

Bicycling. Turn on your back. Raise one knee up to your chest. Then lower it and raise the other knee at the same time. (Feel how the abdominal muscles become tight).

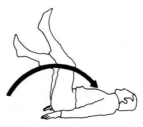

Twisting. Bend both knees as much as you can, your feet flat on the surface; let the knees fall together to one side while keeping your back flat. Repeat on the other side.

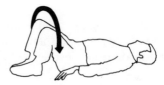

Knee Spreading. From the same position with bent knees, let them fall away from each other. When the knees are wide open, the soles of the feet are flat against each other. Relax while you keep this position three minutes.

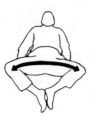

Rolling. Raise your *right* arm over your head and reach up as far as you can while reaching down with your *right* heel; keep up the stretch and roll to your *left* side. Return on your back. Do the same with the other side.

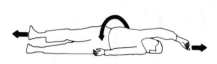

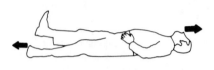

Stretching. Flat on your back, stretch yourself from head to feet, reaching down the bed with the heel (not toes) as far as you can; left heel, then right heel.

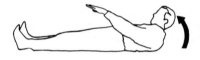

Chest Raising. Flat on back, legs straight, *in*hale deeply. Then, while you *ex*hale, pull your abdomen in, lift your head for one second and return it slowly to the pillow while continuing to exhale. (With increasing training, prolong your expiration and lift head and shoulders. After practice you might try to lift head, shoulders, chest and entire trunk to sitting position).

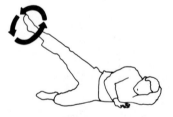

Leg Circling. Lie on your left side, make a circle with your right foot: forward, up and back, keeping the knee straight. Repeat on the other side.

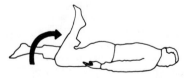

Breathing and Knee Bending. Face down, arms to side, breathe twice deeply, feeling how your back bulges from the inhaled air. Bend knees alternately, trying to get heel close to the buttock.

Sitting Up Exercises

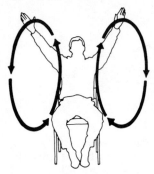

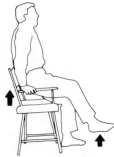

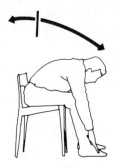

Arm Circling. Raise your arms forward and upward as high as you can, then open them wide and return them to the side. Reverse the motion.

Pushup. (This exercise needs a wheelchair or chair with armrests). Hands on armrests. Push down on your hands, so that your elbows straighten, lifting your entire trunk and raising your buttocks off the seat. Then take one foot off the ground.

Trunk Bending. Stretch your back while you bend your trunk forward with your arms down. Go as far as you can, but only if there is no dizziness, redness of face or other discomfort. Then bend your trunk backward, and to either side.

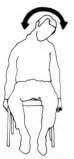

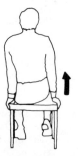

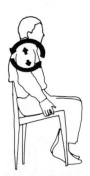

Neck Bending. Now stretch in particular your neck, without raising your chin. While you keep up the stretch of the neck, bend it forward, bringing your chin to your chest. Then bend it backward, then to one side and the other side.

Hip Hiking. Lift one buttock after the other up from the chair, without moving your head away.

Shoulder Circling. Shrug your shoulders and continue their motion backward, downward and forward to a full circle.

NOTE: Do not change directions fast and go very slowly, avoiding dizziness. It is also good not to do all neck bending exercises together but rather to intersperse them among the other exercises. (This applies to all exercises which might result in dizziness, particularly head circling, trunk circling and — more than any other — breathing exercises).

Standing Exercises

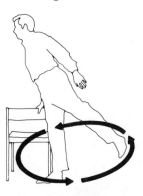

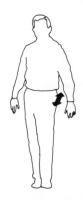

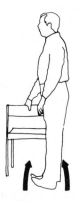

Lower Limb Swinging. While you hold on to a piece of furniture with one or both hands, swing one leg forward and backward; then sideward from left to right; then circle the limb. Try to increase these motions gradually. The motions that count are those in the hip joint.

Pelvic Twisting. With feet together, move one side of your pelvis forward, then the other side, with as little motion as possible of the knees or the shoulders.

Toe and Heel Raising. 1. Raise yourself on your toes. 2. Come down on your heels. 3. Resting on your heels, raise both toes and feet.

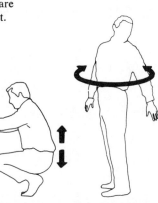

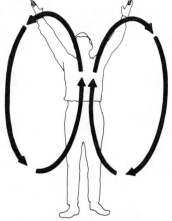

Knee Bending. Take a secure support with both hands and make a knee bend which you make deeper according to your comfort. If you can, do this exercise in two ways: on your toes as well as on the entire sole of the foot.

Trunk Twisting. With legs apart, turn trunk to one side, as if you want to see what is behind you. Then turn to the other side. Keep your pelvis straight while you twist your trunk.

Arm Circling. Stand comfortably. With each arm make a circle which gradually increases to become as large as possible. Do this with both arms at the same time, first in one direction then in the other.

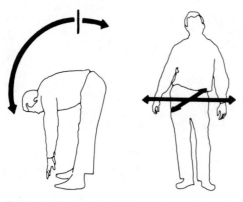

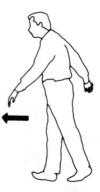

Trunk Bending. Stand securely with your legs about two feet apart. Bend your trunk forward, then backward, then to each side. Go very slowly and stop before getting dizzy.

Pelvic Tilting. With feet slightly apart, move your pelvis from side to side, then forward and backward. Try not to move your shoulders.

Walking and Jogging. You can do this indoors or outdoors. Walk easily, first slowly, then briskly, and add a few jogging steps if you are ready. The feet roll off from heel to toe.

After this workout you should feel refreshed, not exhausted. How you feel will be your guide as to how much to exercise the following day and how much of other activities you may undertake (golfing, bicycling, dancing, or whatever pleases you).

APPENDIX **F** | Exercises for Improving the Circulation

A series of very simple exercises for the lower limbs are the following: dorsiflexion, plantar flexion, inversion and eversion of the feet, extension- abduction and flexion-adduction of the toes.

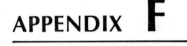

Buerger-Allen Exercises are performed in three stages:

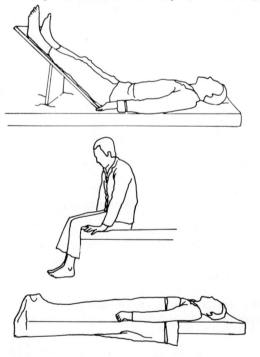

1. Elevation of legs at 45°, propped up by a board or by pillows, is performed until blanching of the feet occurs (about 2 minutes).

2. Immediately thereafter the patient dangles his legs at the edge of the bed, performing exercises of toes and feet in various directions for one to three minutes.

3. The 5-minute rest period that follows is used for warming of the extremities with blanket and heating pad.

From *Exercises for the Elderly* by Herman L. Kamenetz, M.D., a service manual made available by Armour Pharmaceutical Company. Copyright 1971 by Scicom, Inc., Stamford, Connecticut.

219

APPENDIX **G** | Breathing Exercises for Home Use

Your physician has given you this booklet of breathing exercises so that you can help yourself breathe more efficiently. These exercises are designed to train your abdominal muscles to assist your diaphragm in some of the work of breathing. As you get accustomed to this different kind of breathing, you can expect to feel better and be more active in daily life.

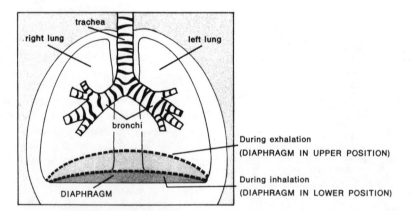

Your physician has checked the exercises that are best for you at this time. The schedule of exercises may change as your new breathing techniques develop. Follow your physician's advice—and remember that the benefit you get from these exercises depends on the regularity and care with which you do them.

Reprinted by permission of Breon Laboratories, Inc.

PREPARATION

Breathing exercises are usually performed two to four times daily: on arising, before meals, during the late afternoon or just before retiring. Each exercise period should last from one-half to one hour, depending on your physician's directions.

Before beginning your exercises, remove tight or restrictive clothing. Be sure your nasal passages are clear. If prescribed by your physician, inhale an aerosol medication according to his directions. This will relax and open the airways in your lungs, and will loosen tenacious mucus so it can be more easily expectorated.

Most important, do not hurry your breathing exercises. Rest when necessary. Do each as long as instructed. And in all cases, begin your day with the BASIC MORNING EXERCISE as shown on page two of this booklet.

AT-HOME BREATHING EXERCISES

Begin exercise sessions with aerosol medication as prescribed by your physician

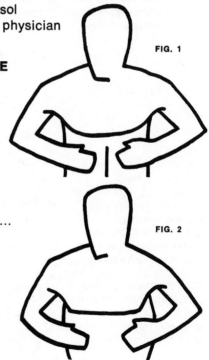

FIG. 1

☐ BASIC MORNING EXERCISE

Sit erect on edge of bed or chair and place hands over lower ribs and upper abdomen as shown in Figure 1. Keep shoulders down, elbows straight out, fingers rigid. Repeat exercise 10 times, or as physician directs.

FIG. 1

EXHALE while applying firm pressure against ribs and abdomen with hands. Exhale slowly through pursed lips... lips held partly open as when you are about to whistle.

FIG. 2

FIG. 2

INHALE after releasing pressure of hands slightly, but still applying effort against chest and abdomen. Cough gently to raise mucus.

▱ EXERCISE ONE

INHALE

EXHALE

Lie flat on floor (*not* on bed) as shown, and rest left hand across chest, right hand on abdomen. Inhale deeply through nose, letting abdomen rise. Then breathe out through pursed lips, pressing inward and upward firmly on abdomen. Try to move the chest as little as possible, letting the abdomen move up and down as you inhale and exhale. As your physician directs, you may practice this exercise while sitting or standing. Repeat 6-8 times. Once you have developed this technique you should breathe in this manner even while walking.

▱ EXERCISE TWO

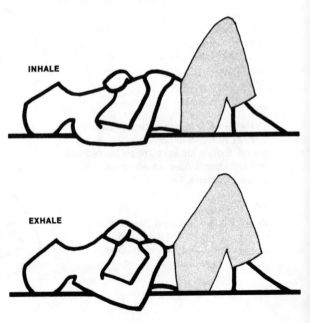

INHALE

EXHALE

Lie flat on floor as shown, and rest left hand across chest, right hand on abdomen. Bend knees, keeping them together. Keep feet on floor, bringing thighs toward chest as far as possible. Inhale through nose, letting abdomen rise. Then breathe out through pursed lips, pressing inward and upward firmly on abdomen. Repeat 6-8 times, or as physician directs.

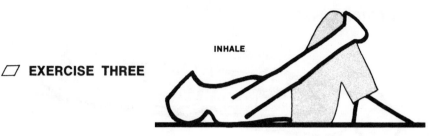

INHALE

▱ EXERCISE THREE

Lie flat on floor as shown, raise
knees and lock arms around legs.
Inhale through nose, letting abdomen
rise. Lift feet from floor and exhale
through pursed lips, pulling legs
toward chest as far as possible with
arms. Repeat 6-8 times, or as
physician directs.

EXHALE

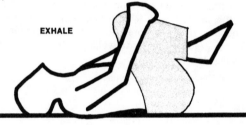

▱ EXERCISE FOUR

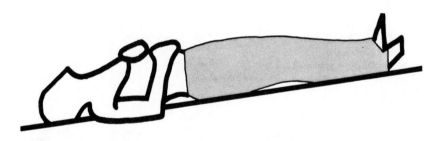

With feet elevated about 14 inches and body in a straight line as shown in
illustration, rest left hand across chest, right hand on abdomen. Inhale deeply
through nose, letting abdomen rise. Then breathe out through pursed lips,
pressing inward and upward firmly on the abdomen. Try to move the chest as
little as possible, letting the abdomen move up and down as you inhale and
exhale. Repeat 6-8 times, or as physician directs.

⟍⟋ EXERCISE FIVE

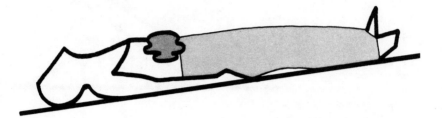

With feet elevated about 14 inches and body in a straight line as shown in illustration, place a five pound weight on the abdomen. (Use rubber hot-water bottle, or cloth sack filled with sand.) Inhale deeply through nose, letting abdomen rise. Then breathe out through pursed lips. Physician may instruct you to gradually increase weight to 15 pounds. Repeat exercise 6-8 times, or as physician directs.

H

Postural
Drainage
Exercises

When mucus accumulates in your lungs, it can thicken and form "plugs" that block small airways and make breathing difficult. Postural drainage is simply a way of letting gravity help you clear out these plugs and mucus, and get them to the mouth where they can be expectorated.

Your Doctor will check the exercises that are best for you. Follow his instructions exactly—and remember that the benefit you get from these exercises depends on the regularity and care with which you do them.

PREPARATION: Postural drainage exercises are usually performed four times a day—on arising, before lunch and dinner, and before bedtime. Follow your Doctor's instructions regarding schedule.

Before beginning your exercises, remove tight or restrictive clothing and wear comfortable trousers or pyjamas. If prescribed by your Doctor, inhale an aerosol medication according to his directions. This will relax and open the airways in your lungs, and loosen tenacious mucus and plugs so they will drain more easily. In addition, your doctor may recommend a chest-tapping procedure that you or an assistant (such as a family member) can use to help dislodge mucus.

In exercises where it is recommended that the foot of the bed be elevated, you may find it most practical to use a lightweight folding canvas cot, which can easily be propped up to the desired height.

Do your exercises in the order your Doctor recommends. Keep a bowl available for the draining mucus. Cover your pillow with a towel to prevent soiling. Do not hurry —hold each position as long as required. And *in all cases,* finish your exercise with the BASIC POSITION as shown on page four of this manual.

Reprinted by permission of Breon Laboratories, Inc.

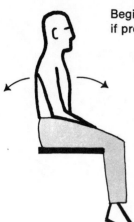

Begin exercise session with aerosol medication if prescribed by your doctor.

EXERCISE 1

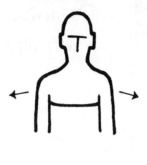

Sit upright on edge of bed or chair, lean slightly back, forward, left and right. Hold each position half a minute.

EXERCISE 2

Lie on back, with small rolled blanket or cushion (6 inches thick) under hips. Bend knees, pull thighs toward chest. Keep feet on bed. Hold position for half a minute.

Note: Foot of bed may be elevated 18 inches for greater effectiveness.

EXERCISE 3

Lie flat on back without pillow, arms at side. Hold position half a minute.

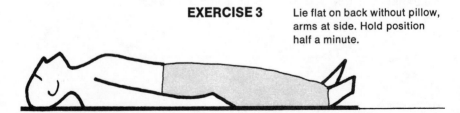

EXERCISE 4

Lie face downward, head on arms, with small rolled blanket or cushion (6 inches thick) under lower abdomen. Hold position half a minute.

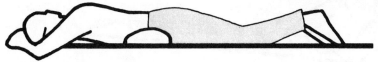

EXERCISE 5

Lie on right side with pillow supporting head, as shown. Hold half a minute. Then swing left shoulder forward, using right shoulder as a pivot. Hold half a minute.

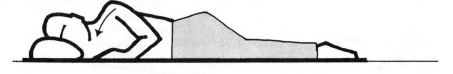

EXERCISE 6

Lie on left side with pillow supporting head, as shown. Hold half a minute. Then swing right shoulder forward, using left shoulder as a pivot. Hold half a minute.

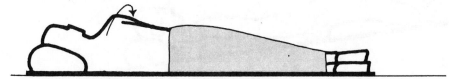

EXERCISE 7   With foot of bed elevated 18 inches, lie on right side. Place small rolled blanket or cushion (6 inches thick) between hip bone and bottom rib. Hold position half a minute.

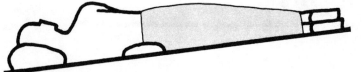

EXERCISE 8   With foot of bed elevated 18 inches, lie on left side. Place small rolled blanket or cushion (6 inches thick) between hip bone and bottom rib. Hold position half a minute.

EXERCISE 9   With foot of bed elevated 18 inches, lie on back, with pillow under knees. Hold position half a minute.

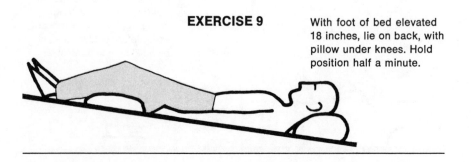

EXERCISE 10   With foot of bed elevated 18 inches, lie on back, with body turned slightly onto left side, pillow under knees. Hold half a minute. Then turn body slightly onto right side. Hold half a minute.

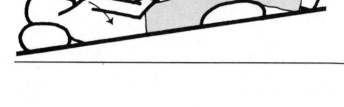

BASIC POSITION   Use this at end of all postural drainage exercises. Lie face down across a level bed, hips at edge of bed. Hold position for 20 to 30 minutes. Rest forearms on floor, forehead on upturned hands. Breathe deeply and cough gently to expel mucus and secretions raised by previous exercises. A folded towel may be used to make forehead and arms more comfortable. Have a bowl available to receive draining mucus.

Suggested Readings

BOOKS AND PAMPHLETS

American Medical Association, Council on Drugs. *AMA Drug Evaluations*. Chicago: American Medical Association, 1971.

App, R. J. *Making the Later Years Count: For a Healthy, Well-Provided, Blessed Old Age*. Milwaukee: Bruce Publishing Company, 1960.

Armour Pharmaceutical Company. *Extended Care in the Home*. Chicago: Armour Pharmaceutical Company, 1972.

Armour Pharmaceutical Company. *Recreation in Golden Age*. Chicago: Armour Pharmaceutical Company, 1972.

Armour Pharmaceutical Company. *What Makes Old Folks Cranky and How to Cope with It*. Chicago: Armour Pharmaceutical Company, 1971.

Beatty, R. P. *The Senior Citizen*. Springfield, Ill.: Charles C Thomas, 1962.

Beeson, P. B. and McDermott, W., Eds. *Cecil-Loeb Textbook of Medicine*, 13th ed. Philadelphia: W. B. Saunders Company, 1971.

Blumberg, J. E. and Drummond, E. E. *Nursing Care of the Long-Term Patient*, 2d ed. New York: Springer Publishing Company, 1971.

Bortz, E. L. *Creative Aging*. New York: The Macmillan Company, 1962.

Botwinick, J. *Cognitive Processes in Maturity and Old Age*. New York: Springer Publishing Company, 1967.

Botwinick, J. *Aging and Behavior*. New York: Springer Publishing Company, 1974.

Boyd, W. *Textbook of Pathology*, 8th ed. Philadelphia: Lea and Febiger, 1970.

Brainerd, H. et al. *Current Diagnosis and Treatment*, 12th ed. Los Altos, Ca.: Lange Medical Publications, 1970.

Breon Laboratories, Inc. *Postural Exercises* (pamphlet). New York: Breon Laboratories, Inc., 1967.

Breon Laboratories, Inc. *Breathing Exercises for Home Use* (pamphlet). New York: Breon Laboratories, Inc., 1970.

Brunner, L. S. and Suddarth, D. S. *The Lippincott Manual of Nursing Practice*. Philadelphia: J. B. Lippincott Company, 1974.

Campbell, M. F. and Harrison, J. H., Eds. *Urology*, 3d ed. Philadelphia: W. B. Saunders Company, 1970.

Conn, H. F., Ed. *Current Therapy*. Philadelphia: W. B. Saunders Company, 1975.

Conn, H. F. et al. *Family Practice*. Philadelphia: W. B. Saunders Company, 1973.

Conn, H. F. and Conn, R. B., Jr., Eds. *Current Diagnosis*. Philadelphia: W. B. Saunders Company, 1975.

Davidshohn, I. and Henry, J. B., Eds. *Todd-Sanford Clinical Diagnosis by Laboratory Methods*, 15th ed. Philadelphia: W. B. Saunders Company, 1974.

Douthwaite, A. H., Ed. *French's Index of Differential Diagnosis*. Baltimore: Williams & Wilkins, 1960.

Durham, R. H., Ed. *Encyclopedia of Medical Syndromes*. New York: Harper and Row, 1962.

Falconer, M. W. et al. *Current Drug Handbook 1976-1978*. Philadelphia: W. B. Saunders Company, 1976.

Goodman, B. L. and Gilman, A. *The Pharmaceutical Basis of Therapeutics*, 3d ed. New York: The Macmillan Company, 1966.

Gordon, B. L. et al. *Current Medical Terminology*, 4th ed. Chicago: American Medical Association, 1971.

Guyton, A. C. *Function of the Human Body*, 4th ed. Philadelphia: W. B. Saunders Company, 1974.

Hazell, K. *Social and Medical Problems of the Elderly*, 3d ed. Springfield, Ill.: Charles C Thomas, 1973.

Howe, P. S. *Basic Nutrition in Health and Disease*, 5th ed. Philadelphia: W. B. Saunders Company, 1971.

Jablonski, S. *Illustrated Dictionary of Eponymic Syndromes and Their Synonyms*. Philadelphia: W. B. Saunders Company, 1969.

Kamenetz, H. L. *A Guide to Geriatric Rehabilitation* (pamphlet). Chicago: Armour Pharmaceutical Company, 1971.

Kastenbaum, R. *New Thoughts on Old Age.* New York: Springer Publishing Company, 1964.

Kastenbaum, R. and Aisenberg, R. *The Psychology of Death.* New York: Springer Publishing Company, 1972.

Kimmig, J. and Janner, M. *Frieboes Schonfeld Color Atlas of Dermatology.* Translated by H. Goldschmidt. Philadelphia: W. B. Saunders Company, 1966.

Kraus, R. *Therapeutic Recreation Services: Principles and Practices.* Philadelphia: W. B. Saunders Company, 1973.

Kübler-Ross, E. K. *On Death and Dying.* New York: The Macmillan Company, 1970.

Lily Research Laboratory. *Diabetes Mellitus,* 7th ed. Indianapolis: The Eli Lily Company, 1967.

Lucas, C. *Recreational Activity Development for the Aging in Homes, Hospitals, and Nursing Homes.* Springfield, Ill.: Charles C Thomas, 1974.

Miller, B. G. and Keane, C. B. *Encyclopedia and Dictionary of Medicine and Nursing.* Philadelphia: W. B. Saunders Company, 1972.

Rosenfeld, M. G., Ed. *Manual of Medical Therapeutics,* 20th ed. Boston: Little, Brown and Company, 1971.

Rudolph, M. and Mueller, C. G. *Light and Vision.* New York: Time-Life Company, 1972.

Sabiston, D. C., Jr. *Davis-Christopher Textbook of Surgery,* 10th ed. Philadelphia: W. B. Saunders Company, 1972.

Thorek, P. *Surgical Diagnosis,* 2d ed. Philadelphia: J. B. Lippincott Company, 1965.

The Upjohn Company. *Diabetes Mellitus—A Collection of Monographs.* n.d.

Vaughan, D. and Asbury, T. *General Ophthalmology,* 7th ed. Los Altos, Ca.: Lange Medical Publications, 1974.

Vedder, C. B., Ed. *Problems of the Middle-Aged.* Springfield, Ill.: Charles C Thomas, 1965.

Whitehead, J. A. *Psychiatric Disorders of Old Age: A Handbook for the Clinical Team.* New York: Springer Publishing Company, 1974.

1971 White House Conference on Aging. *Toward a National Policy on Aging.* Washington, D. C.: U.S. Government Printing Office, 1972.

PERIODICALS

American Journal of Nursing. Nurse practitioners in geriatrics. *American Journal of Nursing* 72:12, pp. 2054-2055, December 1973.

Anagnostopoulis, C. E., et al. Symposium on coronary heart disease. *Medical Clinics of North America* 57:1, January 1973.

Altschule, M. D. Symposium on atherosclerosis. *Medical Clinics of North America* 58:2, pp. 243-244, March 1974.

Archer, S. K. Health maintenance programs for older adults. *Nursing Clinics of North America* 3:4, pp. 725-729, December 1968.

Barnes, B. O., Ratzenhofer, M., and Gisi, R. The role of natural consequences in the changing death patterns. *Journal of the American Geriatric Society* 22:4, pp. 176-179, April 1974.

Barrocos, A. The dying patient—a team affair. *Nursing Digest* 2:5, pp. 62-66, May 1974.

Bayne, J. R. Geriatrics and gerontology in medical education. *Journal of the American Geriatric Society* 22:5, pp. 298-302, May 1974.

Black, Sister Kathleen. Social isolation and the nursing process. *Nursing Clinics of North America* 8:4, pp. 575-586, December 1973.

Branson, F. K. For the geriatric patient the "home away from home" is a myth. *Hospital Management* 98:8, p. 118, August 1964.

Burnside, I. M. Touching is talking. *American Journal of Nursing* 73:12, pp. 2060-2061, December 1973.

Burnside, I. M. Baroque pearls (poem). *American Journal of Nursing* 73:12, p. 2061, December 1973.

Calloway, N. O. Heat production and senescence. *Journal of the American Geriatric Society* 22:4, pp. 149-150, April 1974.

Carmichael, J. and Linn, M. W. Functioning of the elderly patient in relation to the physician's diagnosis of chronic brain syndrome. *Journal of the American Geriatric Society* 22:5, pp. 217-221, May 1974.

Davis, R. W. Psychological aspects of geriatric nursing. *American Journal of Nursing* 68:4, pp. 802-804, April 1974.

DeBakey, M. E. Cardiovascular disorders. *Postgraduate Medicine* 55:3, p. 139, March 1974.

Domming, J. J., Stackman, J., and O'Neill, P., et al. Experiences with dying patients. *American Journal of Nursing* 73:6, pp. 1058-1064, June 1973.

Dorsey, F. G. Adequate hospital care for the aged. *Journal of the American Geriatric Society* 22:4, pp. 180-182, April 1974.

Drummond, E. E. Communication and comfort for the dying patient. *Nursing Clinics of North America* 5:1, p. 55, March 1970.

Elder, R. Dying in the U.S.A. *Nursing Digest* 2:5, pp. 2-11, May 1974.

Elwood, E. Nursing the patient with a cerebrovascular accident. *Nursing Clinics of North America* 5:1, pp. 47-50, March 1970.

Evangela, Sister M. The influence of family relationships on the geriatric patient—the nurse's role. *Nursing Clinics of North America* 3:4, pp. 653-659, September 1968.

Falk, M. A. Treatment of the depressed outpatient. *Postgraduate Medicine* 55:3, pp. 77-81, March 1974.

Farmer, R. G. Anemia: gastrointestinal causes. *Postgraduate Medicine* 52:4, p. 95, October 1972.

Fletcher, J. Ethics and euthanasia. *American Journal of Nursing* 73:4, pp. 670-675, April 1973.

Gaspard, N. J. The family of the patient with long-term illness. *Nursing Clinics of North America* 5:4, p. 7, March 1970.

Geriatric Focus. Latest findings in the biology of aging. *Geriatric Focus* 11:3, p. 1, October 1972.

Geriatric Focus. Long-term care of aged called a "national priority." *Geriatric Focus* 11:3, pp. 1, 7, October 1972.

Geriatric Focus. Group psychotherapy in old age—chance for creative intervention. *Geriatric Focus* 11:4, p. 4, November 1972.

Geriatric Focus. A profile in discouragement: the health crisis now facing elderly people in our inner cities. *Geriatric Focus* 12:1, pp. 2-3, January 1973.

Geriatric Focus. Community care for the impaired elderly as an effective alternative to institutional care. *Geriatric Focus* 12:3, pp. 2-3, March 1973.

Geriatric Focus. Nurses play a vital role in project providing home maintenance for chronically ill aged. *Geriatric Focus* 12:4, pp. 2-3, April 1973.

Geriatric Focus. "Senility" symptoms mask for nutritional deficiencies. *Geriatric Focus* 12:4, pp. 2-3, April 1973.

Geriatric Focus. The opinions and attitudes of nursing home officials. *Geriatric Focus* 12:4, pp. 1, 4-5, April 1973.

Geriatric Focus. Ambivalence in attitudes toward aging and dying. *Geriatric Focus* 12:6, pp. 1, 5-6, June 1973.

Geriatric Focus. Does old age make sense? Not if we regard it as a total calamity, decrepit and demented. *Geriatric Focus* 12:6, pp. 2-3, June 1973.

Geriatric Focus. Doctor/patient relationship: partners in dying. *Geriatric Focus* 12:7, pp. 1, 5-7, July-August, 1973.

Geriatric Focus. A rating scale to determine the type of care best suited to the needs of aged mental patients. *Geriatric Focus* 12:9, pp. 2-3, October 1973.

Geriatric Focus. Social interactions with peers improves functioning health. *Geriatric Focus* 12:10, p. 5, November 1973.

Geriatric Focus. Who's afraid of death? Elderly and religious subjects less afraid than others. *Geriatric Focus* 12:10, pp. 2-3, November 1973.

Goldberg, S. B. Family tasks and functions in the crisis of death. *Nursing Digest* 2:5, pp. 21-26, May 1974.

Gordon, E. S. Diabetes mellitus: new developments. *Postgraduate Medicine* 55:3, pp. 145-149, March 1974.

Greenberg, B. Reaction time in the elderly. *American Journal of Nursing* 73:12, pp. 2056-2058, December 1973.

Hanlan, A. F. Notes of a dying professor. *Nursing Digest* 2:5, pp. 36-42, May 1974.

Harris, R. S., et al. Long-term oral administration of probocol in the management of hypercholesterolemia. *Journal of the American Geriatric Society* 22:4, pp. 167-175, April 1974.

Harrison, C. The institutionally-deprived elderly, a challenge for nurses to change their role. *Nursing Clinics of North America* 3:4, p. 697, December 1968.

Hoffman, E. Carcinoma of the thyroid in patients aged 50 or older. *Journal of the American Geriatric Society* 22:4, pp. 151-166, April 1974.

Hulicka, I. M. Fostering self-respect in aged patients. *American Journal of Nursing* 64:4, pp. 84-86, March 1964.

Human, M. E. Death of a neighbor. *American Journal of Nursing* 73:11, pp. 1914-1916, November 1973.

Irwin, T. How to handle problems of aging. *Today's Health* 47:7, pp. 28-31, February 1969.

Isler, C. Decubitus/old truths and some new ideas. *RN* 35:7, pp. 42-45, July 1972.

Jousey, J., et al. Newer concepts in the treatment of osteoporosis. *Postgraduate Medicine* 54:2, p. 62, October 1972.

Kamenetz, H. L. Exercises for the elderly. *American Journal of Nursing* 72:8, p. 1401, August 1972.

Kavanaugh, R. E. Helping patients who are facing death. *Nursing '74* 4:5, pp. 35-42, May 1974.

Knudson, R. J. and Burrows, B. Early detection of obstructive lung disease. *Medical Clinics of North America* 57:3, pp. 681-690, May 1973.

Knowles L. N., Ed. Symposium on putting geriatric nursing standards into practice. *Nursing Clinics of North America* 72:6, p. 201, June 1972.

Koenig, R. Dying vs well-being. *Nursing Digest* 2:5, pp. 49-50, May 1974.

Lane, H. C. et al., Eds. Symposium on care of the elderly patient. *Nursing Clinics of North America* 3:4, pp. 649-651 (Foreword), December 1968.

MacRae, I. Arthritis, its nature and management. *Nursing Clinics of North America* 8:4, pp. 643-652, December 1973.

Mervyn, F. The plight of the dying patient in the hospital. *American Journal of Nursing* 71:5, pp. 1988-1990, May 1971.

Miller, P. G. and Ozga, J. "Mommy, what happens when I die?" *Nursing Digest* 2:5, pp. 76-79, May 1974.

Modell, W., et al. Symposium on use of drugs in the elderly patient. *Medical Clinics of North America* 29:6, June 1974.

Morris, M. M. and Rhoads, M. Guidelines for the care of confused patients. *American Journal of Nursing* 72:9, pp. 1630-1634, September 1972.

Ornstein, S. Objective—a national policy on aging. *American Journal of Nursing* 71:5, pp. 960-963, May 1971.

Patrick, M. L. Care of the confused elderly patient. *American Journal of Nursing* 67:12, pp. 2536-2539, December 1967.

Penalver, M. Death watch (poem). *American Journal of Nursing* 73:11, p. 1916, November 1973.

Preston, T. When words fail. *American Journal of Nursing* 73:12, pp. 2064-2066, December 1973.

Quilitch, H. R. Purposeful activity increased on a geriatric ward through programmed recreation. *Journal of the American Geriatric Society* 22:5, pp. 226-229, May 1974.

Ray, A. K. and Rao, D. B. Calcium metabolism in elderly epileptic patients during anticonvulsant therapy. *Journal of the American Geriatric Society* 22:5, pp. 222-225, May 1974.

Rhoades, F. P. Continuous cyclic hormonal therapy. *Journal of the American Geriatric Society* 22:4, p. 183, April 1974.

Richards, B. An old man's prayer (poem). *American Journal of Nursing* 73:4, p. 675, April 1974.

Roberts, J. L. and Kimsey, L. R. How does it feel to grow old? *Nursing Digest* 1:8, p. 24, October 1973.

Robison, S. Home visits to the elderly. *American Journal of Nursing* 74:5, pp. 908-909, May 1974.

Rodstein, M. Health problems of the aged. *RN* 35:8, pp. 39-43, August 1972.

Ross, C. H. Geriatrics and the elderly woman. *Journal of the American Geriatric Society* 22:5, pp. 230-239, May 1974.

Rubin, A. D., et al. Symposium on clinical diagnosis of blood diseases. *Medical Clinics of North America* 57:2, p. 253, March 1973.

Schwab, Sister Marilyn. Caring for the aged, Part I. *American Journal of Nursing* 73:12, pp. 2049-2053, December 1973.

Schultz, L. C. Nursing care of the stroke patient—rehabilitative aspects. *Nursing Clinics of North America* 8:4, pp. 633-642, December 1973.

Scott, M. L. To learn to live with the elderly. *American Journal of Nursing* 73:4, pp. 662-664, April 1973.

Soika, C. V. Combatting osteoporosis. *American Journal of Nursing* 73:7, pp. 1193-1197, July 1973.

Stewart, S. Looking back (poem). *American Journal of Nursing* 73:12, p. 2059, December 1973.

Swanburg, H. and Snively, W. D. Geriatrics, food for thought. *Abbotempe* 3:4, p. 20, April 1965.

Todd, R. L. Early treatment reverses symptoms of senility. *Hospital and Community Psychiatrist* 7:16, pp. 170-171, June 1966.

Toussie, A. G. "Mabel, you don't belong here." *American Journal of Nursing* 73:12, p. 2059, December 1973.

Tuck, R. R. The geriatric nurse, pioneer of a new specialty. *RN* 35:8, pp. 35-38, August 1972.

Vavrid, M. "High risk" factors and atherosclerotic cardiovascular diseases of the aged. *Journal of the American Geriatric Society* 22:5, p. 203, May 1973.

Volpe, A. and Kastenbaum, R. Beer and TLC. *American Journal of Nursing* 67:1, pp. 100-103, January 1967.

Walker, M. The last hour before death. *American Journal of Nursing* 73:9, pp. 1592-1593, September 1973.

Weber, L. J. Ethics and euthanasia: another view. *American Journal of Nursing* 73:7, pp. 1228-1231, July 1973.

Weymouth, L. T. The nursing care of the so-called confused patient. *Nursing Clinics of North America* 3:4, pp. 709-715, December 1968.

Glossary

abort   to check a disease process in its early stages.

abrasion   a break in the skin or mucous membrane caused by rubbing or scraping.

abscess   a localized collection of pus formed by the disintegration of tissue by the action of bacteria.

acidosis   depletion of the body's alkali reserve with resulting disturbance of the acid-base balance.

acquired   not inherited.

acute   short and severe; not drawn out over a long period of time; the opposite of chronic.

Addison's disease   a condition caused by deficient secretion by the adrenal cortex; manifested by electrolytic upset, lowered blood volume, anemia, muscular weakness, bronzing of the skin.

adenitis   inflammation of a lymph gland or lymph node.

adenocarcinoma   a malignant growth of glandular tissue.

adenoma   a tumor of glandular tissue.

ADH   *see* antidiuretic hormone.

adhesion   the union of two parts that do not belong together; the band of fibrous tissue that joins such parts.

adrenocorticosteroid   a hormone produced by the cortex of the adrenal gland.

agammaglobulinemia   absence of gamma globulin in the blood, with consequent inability to produce immunity to infection.

agnosia   inability to recognize sensory impressions; may refer to vision, hearing, taste, smell, etc.

allergen   any agent that produces a state of allergy; may be protein or nonprotein (for example, hair or fur, drugs, foods, dust, fungi, bacteria, pollens).

allergy   a reaction to a particular allergen or a foreign substance that is harmless to most people.

amblyopia   defective vision when there is no detectable reason for it.

amenorrhea   absence of menstruation.

amnesia   partial or complete loss of memory.

anabolic   refers to the phase of metabolism during which food substances are utilized to form body substances.

analgesic   a drug that relieves pain; insensitivity to pain; having the effect of relieving pain.

anemia   term used to describe a large group of disorders that result from a deficiency of red blood cells or their hemoglobin, or both.

anesthesia   loss of sensation.

aneurysm   a sac-like bulging of a blood vessel wall due to weakening by disease or by a congenital anomaly.

angiogram   x-ray of blood vessels after injection of a radiopaque substance.

ankylosis   stiffening or fixation of a joint.

anomaly   that which is unusual, abnormal, or nonconforming in structure, form, or location.

anorexia   loss or deficiency of appetite for food.

antacid   a substance that neutralizes or counteracts acidity.

anterior   the front surface; in front of.

antianemic   an agent that relieves or counteracts anemia.

anticoagulant   an agent that prevents or retards clotting of the blood.

anticonvulsant   an agent that prevents or stops convulsions.

antidiuretic hormone   a hormone secreted by the pituitary gland; influences the amount of urine secreted.

antiembolic   literally, against embolism. Antiembolic stockings are made of elastic material and applied postoperatively or at other times when there is danger of or tendency to thromboembolism.

antihyperglycemic   an agent that counteracts high levels of glucose (sugar) in the blood.

anti-infective   counteracting infection.

antimetabolite   a substance that replaces or interferes with the body's utilization of an essential compound produced during metabolism.

antineoplastic   an agent that interferes with or prevents the growth of a neoplasm or the spreading of malignant cells in the body.

antitussive   any measure or agent that relieves or suppresses cough.

antrum   a closed or nearly closed cavity, especially in a bone.

anuria   absence of secretion of urine.

anus   the extreme end of the rectum.

apathy   abnormal listlessness and lack of activity.

aphasia   loss or impairment of the ability to use words to express one's thoughts, or impairment of the ability to comprehend written or spoken language.

apical beat   heartbeat heard in the fifth intercostal space in the midclavicular line, the lowest and most lateral point at which an impulse can be detected.

apnea   lack of breathing.

apraxia   loss of ability to perform purposeful movements such as tying shoelaces.

areflexia   the state of being without reflexes.

arteriole   a small artery, particularly one joining an artery to a capillary.

arteriosclerosis   degenerative changes in the arteries, especially a thickening of the walls with loss of elasticity.

arthritis   inflammation of one or more joints, often accompanied by pain, stiffness, and structural changes.

articular   pertaining to a joint.

ascites   the accumulation of free fluid in the peritoneal cavity; sometimes called "abdominal dropsy."

aspiration   the withdrawal of fluid from a body cavity by suction; the act of drawing or inhaling into the lung a foreign substance such as a food particle.

asymptomatic   without symptoms.

asystole   imperfect, incomplete, or absent contraction of the ventricles during the systolic phase of the heartbeat.

ataxia   defective muscular control resulting in jerky and irregular movements, due to a lesion in the central nervous system.

ataxic gait   the foot is raised high and then brought down suddenly, the whole foot striking the ground.

atelectasis   partial or complete collapse of the lung.

atheroma   a mass of fatty yellow substance deposited in the wall of a blood vessel; atheromatous is the adjective.

atherosclerosis   a condition in which the inner layer of the artery wall becomes thickened due to deposits of foreign material, usually a fatty substance.

atopic   refers to a form of allergy or hypersensitivity such as hay fever or asthma.

atrophy   wasting, emaciation, or diminution in size and function of an organ or part that had previously reached mature size.

atypical   unusual, irregular, not typical.

audiometry   measurement of the acuteness of one's hearing.

aura   a premonition or a peculiar sensation or warning that is recognized by the patient.

auscultation   a method of listening to body sounds for diagnostic purposes, particularly the heart, lungs, fetal circulation; the examiner's ear or a stethoscope may be used.

auscultatory   refers to a method of examination that involves listening to body sounds by ear or with a stethoscope.

automatism   performance of involuntary acts without intent or purpose.

autophony   the sensation that one's voice is abnormally loud.

axilla   the armpit.

azotemia   the presence of pathological amounts of nitrogenous products, especially urea, in the blood.

bacillus   a general term used to designate any rod-shaped microorganism.

bacteremia   presence of bacteria in the blood.

barium enema   an enema of barium given before examination of the lower intestinal tract; it is retained while the colon is examined under a fluoroscope and x-ray films are taken.

basal ganglia   four small islands of gray matter located in the white matter at the base of the cerebrum.

basal metabolic rate   the rate at which energy is expended by a person at complete physical rest.

benign   innocent; mild; the opposite of malignant.

bilateral   having or pertaining to two sides.

biliary   pertaining to bile, the bile ducts, or the gallbladder.

biopsy   term used to describe removal of tissue from a living body for examination to establish a diagnosis.

bleb   a large blister.

BMR   basal metabolic rate.

bradycardia   slow rate of heart contraction resulting in a slow pulse rate.

brain scan   a visual examination of a small area of the brain in great detail.

broad-spectrum drug   usually refers to an antibiotic drug that is effective against several kinds of bacteria.

bronchiectasis   chronic dilatation of the bronchi, characterized by productive cough, profuse expectoration of material consisting of mucus and pus, foul breath, and enlargement of the air passages.

bronchoalveolitis   bronchopneumonia.

bronchodilator   an agent that causes dilatation of the bronchi, thus increasing the caliber of the air passages.

bronchopneumonia   inflammation of the bronchi and lungs; caused by a number of microorganisms or may be secondary to other disease such as measles, whooping cough, or upper respiratory infections.

broncoscopy   examination of the interior of the bronchi with an endoscopic type of instrument.

bruit   a sound or murmur heard by listening with a stethoscope.

bulla   a large watery blister.

bursa   a fibrous sac containing a small amount of fluid; facilitates movement without friction between tendon and bone, skin and bone, and muscle and bone.

bypass surgery   term applied to a surgical procedure that involves a shunt or diversion of blood through other than the usual channel; in open heart surgery it refers to the use of a pump-oxygenator (heart-lung machine) to exclude the heart and lungs from the circulation.

calcific   forming or causing a deposit of lime or other insoluble calcium salt.

calculus   an abnormal concentration of minerals, commonly called a "stone."

carbohydrate   a compound containing carbon, hydrogen, and oxygen, the latter two in proportion to form water; present in most foods, but chiefly in sugars and starches.

carboxyhemoglobin   a stable compound of carbon monoxide and hemoglobin.

carcinoma   a malignant tumor arising from epithelial tissue.

cardiac decompensation   inability of the heart to maintain normal circulation throughout the body.

cardiologist   a physician who is particularly skilled in the treatment of diseases of the heart.

cardiomegaly   enlargement of the heart.

carotid sinus   a slight deviation at the place in the neck where the internal carotid artery branches from the common carotid artery, containing special nerve endings that cause a change in heart rate when stimulated. External pressure on it can result in a drop in blood pressure and faintness.

catalepsy   a conscious but trancelike state in which the muscles are rigid so that the subject remains in a fixed position over an indefinite period of time.

catatonic   refers to a type of behavior in which the person may assume odd postures or positions for indefinite periods of time.

catecholamines   compounds that have the power to cause changes in the body similar to those caused by action of nerves in the sympathetic system.

catheterization   the insertion of a catheter (hollow tube) into a body channel or cavity, usually in the urinary bladder.

cerebral   pertaining to or affecting the cerebrum of the brain.

chemotherapeutic   refers to a chemical agent that is used to eradicate or arrest a specific disease.

chemotherapy   treatment with chemical compounds.

Cheyne-Stokes respirations   breathing characterized by rhythmic increase and decrease in depth of respiration with regularly occurring periods of no breathing.

cholecystitis   inflammation of the gallbladder.

choledocholithiasis   stones (calculi) in the common bile duct.

cholelith   a gallstone.

cholelithiasis   the presence of gallstones.

chondrocalcinosis   pseudo-gout, an apparently hereditary condition resembling gout.

chronic   lingering, lasting; the opposite of acute.

circle of Willis   a pattern of arteries at the base of the brain.

circumscribed   confined to a limited area or space.

cirrhosis   hardening; said of an organ such as the liver.

clavicle   the collarbone.

climacteric   the menopause or "change of life."

clonic   refers to spasms of muscles in which rigidity and relaxation alternate.

coccus   a round-shaped bacterium.

colic   severe pain resulting from a spasm in the abdomen or tubular organ.

colposcopy   examination of the vagina and cervix by means of a lighted instrument called a **colposcope.**

coma   complete loss of consciousness.

complete blood count   a count of all the different kinds of cells in the blood.

complication   an accident or second disease that arises in the course of a primary disease and adds to its severity.

concussion   a condition resulting from a violent jar, blow, or shock; usually refers to the brain.

confabulation   a state of confusion in which there is loss of memory for recent events; the gaps are filled in by stories that the individual invents.

congenital   present at birth and existing from that time.

congestion   abnormal accumulation of fluid (usually blood) in a part or an organ.

conjunctiva   the delicate transparent membrane that lines the inner surface of the eyelids and is reflected over the surface of the eyeballs.

constipation   infrequent and usually difficult bowel movements.

contracture   permanent shortening of muscle or scar tissue, producing a deformity.

contralateral   pertaining to or occurring on the opposite side.

convulsion   violent involuntary contraction of voluntary muscles.

coronary   refers to the arteries that supply the heart muscle with blood.

cor pulmonale   heart disease that results from disease of the lungs or of the blood vessels of the lung.

Corrigan pulse   a pulse that rises abruptly and then falls away; also called waterhammer pulse.

cortex   an outer layer as distinguished from the inner substance of an organ; the cerebral cortex is the outer layer of gray matter that covers the two hemispheres of the cerebrum of the brain.

cortical   refers to the outer layer of an organ; the gray matter of the brain is in this layer.

corticosteroids   substances, some of which are hormones, produced in the cortex of the adrenal glands.

cortisone   one of the principal hormones of the adrenal gland.

cranial vault   the skull.

crepitus   a dry, crackling sound such as might be produced by the grating of the ends of a broken bone.

culture   the cultivation of bacteria or of living cells in an artificial medium.

Cushing's syndrome   the appearance of such symptoms as edema, fatness of the face, neck, and trunk, abnormal distribution of hair, amenorrhea, impotence, and atrophy of the genital organs; due to a disorder of the adrenal cortex.

cutaneous   refers to the skin.

cyanosis   bluish discoloration of the skin and mucous membranes, due to lack of oxygen in the blood cells.

cystitis   inflammation of a bladder, particularly the urinary bladder.

cystocele   prolapse of the posterior wall of the urinary bladder into the anterior vaginal wall.

cystoscopy   examination of the urinary tract with a cystoscope, a lighted tubular instrument.

debilitating   weakening

debilitation   a state of weakness or infirmity.

decompensation   term applied to the condition in which the heart is unable to maintain adequate circulation.

decompression   removal of pressure or of a compressing force.

decongestant   an agent or drug that reduces congestion.

decubitus ulcer   bedsore.

defecation   discharge of feces from the rectum.

degeneration   deterioration.

dehydration   loss or removal of fluid from the body in excess of normal amounts.

delusion   a false belief that cannot be altered by argument or reasoning.

dementia   deterioration of mentality, madness.

depigmentation   loss of pigment, usually in the skin.

depressed skull fracture   a skull fracture in which the broken bone presses on the brain.

dermatitis   inflammation of the skin.

dermatosis   any disorder or disease of the skin.

desquamation   shedding, usually said of the skin or mucous membrane.

diabetes mellitus   a condition in which the body does not metabolize carbohydrates, due to lack of production of insulin by the pancreas.

diagnosis   the decision as to which disease or disorder is present.

diarrhea   frequent, loose bowel movements.

diastole   the period of relaxation of the heart.

diathermy   local elevation of temperature in body tissues through the use of high-frequency electric current.

differential blood count   the determination of the number of the various types of white blood cells in a given sample.

diplopia   double vision.

discrete   separate, not joined together, such as a mass that can be felt as separate from the surrounding tissue.

disease entity   a group of signs and symptoms that are related to a specific condition.

disorientation   loss of awareness of one's position relative to the environment.

disseminated   widely spread or scattered.

diuresis   increased secretion of urine.

diuretic   a drug or agent that increases the flow of urine.

diverticulosis   inflammation of a diverticulum.

diverticulum   a circumscribed pouch or sac protruding from the wall of a tube or hollow organ; occurs chiefly in the intestine.

dorsiflexion   bending backwards of the hand or foot.

duodenum   the first part of the small intestine.

dysarthria   difficulty in articulating words; stammering.

dysfunction   abnormal function.

dysphagia   pain or difficulty in swallowing.

dysphonia   unnatural sound of the voice, such as hoarseness or difficulty in speaking.

dyspnea   difficult or labored breathing.

dysuria   difficult or painful urination.

edema   accumulation of an abnormally large amount of fluid in body tissues; **pitting edema** retains for a time the indentation produced by pressure with a finger.

effusion   escape of fluid into a tissue or cavity of the body.

electrocardiogram   a graphic recording of the electrical current produced by the contraction of heart muscle; abbreviated **ECG** (sometimes **EKG**).

electroconvulsive   refers to a type of therapy that consists of applying an electric current to the brain; therapy is also called electroshock.

electroencephalogram   a graphic record of the electric currents developed by the brain; abbreviated **EEG**.

electrolyte   a liquid or solution of a substance that is capable of conducting electricity and is decomposed by it.

emaciation   excessive thinness or wasting of body tissues.

embolism   sudden obstruction of a blood vessel by gas, a clot, or some other solid body.

embolus   a blood clot floating or moving in the bloodstream.

emphysema   the abnormal presence of gas or air in body tissues; occurs most often in the lungs.

encephalopathy   disease or dysfunction of the brain or any part of it.

endarterectomy   surgical removal of atheromatous plaques from an artery (see **atheroma**).

endarteritis   inflammation of the lining of an artery.

endocarditis   inflammation of the membrane that lines the heart.

endogenous   originating within an organ or structure.

endoscope   a tubular, lighted instrument for visualization of body cavities or organs.

enteric   pertaining to the intestine.

enterocele   hernia of the intestine; can be into the upper part of the vagina (see **hernia**).

enterolith   an intestinal "stone."

epidermoid   of the skin, or resembling the skin.

epigastric   above or over the stomach.

epileptiform   resembling epilepsy.

epistaxis   nosebleed.

erotic   refers to sexual passion or interest; lustful.

erythema   redness or congestion of the skin caused by engorgement of the capillaries in the skin.

erythematous   pertains to reddened skin, with or without the escape of fluid.

erythroderma   excessive redness of the skin.

esophageal varices   varicose veins in the wall of the esophagus.

esophagus   the tube through which food passes from the mouth to the stomach.

estrogen   collective name for the female sex hormones secreted within the ovary.

etiology   the science that deals with the causes of disease.

eunuchoidism   deficiency of testes or testicular secretion that results in impaired sexual power.

exacerbation   a flareup of symptoms that have subsided.

excision   surgical removal of an organ or other part of the body.

excoriation   loss or removal of skin such as that produced by scratching, scraping, burns, or chemicals.

exfoliative   refers to the scaling off of tissues in layers.

exophthalmos   abnormal protrusion of the eyeball.

extravasation   escape of blood, lymph, or fluid from its normal enclosure into the surrounding tissues.

extrinsic   developing or having its origin from without.

exudate   serum and blood cells that have oozed out from capillaries or venules.

fascia   the connective tissue sheath that unites the skin to the underlying tissues.

febrile   feverish.

fecalith   a "stone" formed in the intestine from fecal matter.

feces   waste matter excreted from the bowel.

festination   an involuntary hastening in gait.

fetid   having a foul odor.

fibrinous   like fibrin, an insoluble protein that is necessary for the clotting of blood.

fibrosis   the formation of fibrous tissue in an organ or part; usually part of a reparative process.

fissure   a narrow slit, cleft, or groove.

fistula   an abnormal communication between two body surfaces or cavities or between an internal organ and the surface of the body.

flaccid   soft, flabby, not firm.

flatulence   gastric and/or intestinal distension with gas.

fluoroscopy   x-ray examination by means of a fluorescent screen.

focal   localized.

Fowler's position   position in which the patient's head or the head of the bed is elevated 18 to 20 inches above the level, and the knees are flexed.

fremitus   a vibration or thrill, especially one that is perceived by feeling or listening to chest sounds.

friction rub   a friction sound heard when two inflamed or roughened surfaces rub together.

fulminating   developing quickly and with great severity.

furunculosis   the occurrence of furuncles (boils) on the skin.

gallop rhythm   an extra, distinctly heard heart sound that resembles the sound of a horse's gallop; occurs when the heart rate is rapid.

ganglion   an organized mass of cell bodies outside the brain and spinal cord; plural, ganglia.

gangrene   death of part of the tissues of the body; usually the result of inadequate blood supply.

gastritis   inflammation of the stomach.

gastroscopy   inspection of the interior of the stomach with a lighted instrument.

gerontology   the science that deals with the physical and mental changes that occur with aging.

glossitis   inflammation of the tongue.

glottis   the part of the larynx (windpipe) that is associated with voice production.

glucocorticoid   any steroid hormone which promotes the formation of glucose from glycogen; occurs naturally in the adrenal cortex.

glucose   dextrose or grape sugar; occurs naturally in most fruits; it is also the form in which carbohydrates are absorbed from the intestine.

goiter   enlargement of the thyroid gland causing a swelling in the front of the neck.

gonad   a sex gland (testis in the male, ovary in the female).

gram-negative   term used to describe an organism that does not retain the gram stain but takes the counterstain.

gram-positive   term used to describe a microorganism that retains the gram stain when studied in the laboratory.

granulation   the outgrowth of new capillaries and connective tissue from the surface of an open wound.

granuloma   a tumor formed of granulation tissue.

gynecologist   a physician who specializes in the treatment of diseases peculiar to women.

hair follicle   a tubular, oil-secreting, telescoping place in the skin in which a hair grows.

hallucination   a false perception regarded by the individual as real; may involve vision, hearing, taste, smell, or sense of touch.

hallucinogenic   capable of producing hallucinations.

hebephrenic   a type of schizophrenia characterized by silly, uncoordinated behavior.

hematemesis   the vomiting of blood.

hematocrit   term used to express the percentage volume of red cells in the blood.

hematuria   the presence of blood in the urine.

hemianesthesia   anesthesia (loss of sensation) affecting only one side of the body.

hemianopsia   defective vision or blindness in one half of the field of vision in one or both eyes.

hemiplegia   paralysis of one side of the body.

hemoglobin   the oxygen-carrying coloring matter in red blood cells.

hemoglobinuria   the presence of free hemoglobin in the urine.

hemoptysis   the spitting of blood or blood-tinged mucus.

hemorrhage   the escape of copious amounts of blood from a vessel.

hemorrhoid   a varicose vein in the rectal area.

hepatitis   inflammation of the liver.

hepatomegaly   enlargement of the liver.

hernia   the protrusion of an organ or part through an abnormal opening in the surrounding structures.

herpes   an eruption of blisters, often due to a viral infection.

hiatus   a space or opening.

hirsutism   abnormal growth of hair.

Howship-Romberg sign   sharp, darting, tearing pain in the leg; sign of incarcerated femoral hernia.

hydronephrosis   distension of the pelvis of the kidney with urine; due to obstruction of outflow of urine.

hydrotherapy   treatment of disease by the scientific application of water, hot or cold, externally or internally.

hydroureter   abnormal distension of a ureter with urine.

hyperalgesia   excessive sensitivity to pain.

hypercalcemia   excessive calcium in the blood.

hypercalciuria   excretion of urine that contains an abnormal amount of calcium.

hyperesthesia   excessive sensitiveness of the skin or other sense organ.

hyperestrinism   excessive secretion of an estrogenic hormone, characterized by excessive bleeding.

hyperextension   overextension of a limb or other part of the body.

hyperglycemia   an excessive amount of sugar in the blood.

hyperhydrosis   excessive sweating.

hyperkinetic   excessively active and restless.

hypermotility   excessive movement.

hyperpigmentation   increased or excessive deposit of pigment in any of the body tissues; usually refers to the skin.

hyperplasia   excessive formation of cells resulting in overgrowth of tissue.

hyperpnea   rapid, deep breathing.

hyperreflexia   exaggeration of the reflexes, for example, the knee jerk.

hypersensitivity   a state of undue sensitiveness to a stimulus or an allergen.

hypersplenism   a condition in which the inhibitory or destructive functions of the spleen are exaggerated, resulting in a deficiency of certain blood elements in the peripheral blood.

hypertension   abnormally high blood pressure.

hyperthyroidism   a group of symptoms caused by oversecretion of the thyroid hormone.

hypertrophy   increase in the bulk of a tissue or structure that is not the result of tumor.

hypnotic   sleep-producing.

hypochondria   excessive anxiety about one's health, often involving a fixed idea that an organ or body part is diseased.

hypoglycemia less than the normal amount of sugar (glucose) in the blood.

hypotension usually refers to blood pressure below 100/70 and may be a sign of shock.

hypothermia a condition of being below normal body temperature; may be due to a pathological condition or artificially produced.

hypothyroidism a group of symptoms caused by insufficient secretion of the thyroid hormone.

hypoxemia less than the normal amount of oxygen in the blood.

hysterectomy surgical removal of the uterus.

iatrogenic refers to a secondary condition that arises from treatment for a primary condition.

ichthyosis dryness, roughness, and scaliness of the skin due to hypertrophy of the outer layer of the skin.

icterus jaundice.

idiopathic refers to a condition of unknown or spontaneous origin.

ileus intestinal obstruction due to lack of muscular propulsion (paralysis).

illusion misidentification of a sensation.

impetigo a common, acute, inflammatory disease of the skin characterized by the formation of pustules.

incarceration abnormal imprisonment of a part, as in a hernia.

incision a cut or wound produced by cutting into body tissue.

incontinence inability to control any evacuation, especially of urine or feces.

induration the hardening of tissue.

infarction death of tissue in a localized area because the blood supply has been cut off.

infection condition produced by introduction and growth of bacteria in the body.

infectious capable of being transmitted from one person to another.

infestation invasion of the body by insects such as lice, mites, or ticks.

inflammation reaction of tissues to injury, irritation, or infection; characterized by pain, heat, redness, and swelling.

ingestion the act of taking food, fluid, or other substance into the stomach.

inguinal pertaining to the groin.

inguinal canal a canal in the groin through which the spermatic cord of the male or the round ligament of the female passes.

inoculation the introduction of material for the purpose of creating immunity to a disease by giving the individual a mild case of the disease.

insidious having an imperceptible beginning.

insomnia sleeplessness, especially when chronic.

insulin a secretion of the pancreas that has a profound effect on the metabolism of carbohydrates; prepared commercially for treatment of diabetes mellitus.

intercrural between the legs.

intercurrent intervening; said of a disease that arises in a person already suffering from another disease.

intergluteal between the buttocks.

intermittent occurring at intervals.

internist a physician trained in internal medicine as distinguished from a surgeon.

intervertebral disc a pad of cartilage and fiber enclosing the pulpy masses (nucleus pulposus) that lie between the vertebrae and cushion them by absorbing strain and shock and allowing for various movements of the spine.

intra-articular within a joint.

intractable resistant to treatment; obstinate.

intravenous within a vein or going into a vein.

intrinsic inherent; from within; natural.

introitus an opening or entrance to a cavity, particularly the vagina.

intussusception a telescoping of part of the bowel into an adjoining part, causing an obstruction of the bowel.

ipsilateral pertaining to or occurring on the same side.

irradiation treatment by subjecting the patient to the action of such rays as those of heat, light, radium, etc.

ischemia local temporary anemia of a part.

jaundice yellowness of the skin and eyes caused by an excess of bile pigment in the blood.

jejunum the second part of the small intestine, between the duodenum and the ileum.

kyphoscoliosis both a backward and a lateral curvature of the spine.

kyphosis exaggerated curve of the spine in the thoracic region; humpback.

lacrimation weeping.

larynx the organ of voice situated below the pharynx and above the upper end of the trachea.

lateral away from the midline of the body; at the side.

lavage   washing out of a body cavity.

lesion   any pathological change in the continuity or structure of a tissue, whether caused by injury or disease; includes wounds, sores, ulcers, tumors, eruptions, etc.

leukoplakia   a disease characterized by white, thickened patches on mucous membrane, usually of the lips and inside of the mouth.

leukorrhea   sticky, whitish vaginal discharge containing mucus and pus cells.

lipid   one of a group of naturally occurring substances consisting of fatty acids.

localized   restricted to one area or spot; not spread throughout the body.

lordosis   exaggerated forward (convex) curve of the lumbar spine.

lumbar   pertaining to the loins.

lumen   the channel of a tubular structure.

lung scan   an examination of a small area or several areas of the lung in great detail by a specific photographic method.

lymphadenopathy   any disease of the lymph glands.

lymphedema   swelling of the subcutaneous tissues with excess lymph, caused by faulty lymph drainage.

macular   resembling a macule (stain or discolored spot on the skin that is not elevated).

malaise   a feeling of illness and discomfort.

malignant   virulent and dangerous; refers to a condition or disease that is likely to become progressively worse and to end fatally.

malignant hypertension   hypertension that occurs without observable cause, has a stormy onset and a poor prognosis.

malnutrition   the state of being poorly nourished; caused by insufficient intake of food or lack of essential nutrients in the diet.

mammography   x-ray examination of the breast (with or without injection of an opaque medium), used in diagnosis of cancer and other disorders of the breast.

matrix   the foundation substance in which tissue cells are imbedded.

Meckel's diverticulum   a relic of a fetal structure that remains as an appendage of the intestine near the cecum (see diverticulum).

medulla   any soft, marrowlike structure; for example, the center of long bones, the soft internal part of glands and of such organs as the kidney, or the upper part of the spinal cord.

melancholia an extremely unhappy state; in psychiatry, descriptive of severe forms of depression.

melanin dark brown or black pigment normally found in the skin and hair.

melena the passage of dark, tarry stools (colored by the presence of blood).

meningitis inflammation of the membranes that cover the brain and spinal cord.

menopause the permanent cessation of menstruation.

menorrhagia excessive menstruation.

mesenteric pertains to the mesentery, a large fold of peritoneum that invests the intestines and attaches them to the posterior abdominal wall.

metabolism the series of physical and chemical changes in the body by which the body is nourished, energy is produced, and life is maintained.

metastasis transfer of a disease from the original site to another part of the body, usually by blood or lymph.

metatarsophalangeal referring to the foot and toes.

migratory moving from place to place.

miosis excessive contraction of the pupils.

miotic a drug that contracts the pupils.

monocular pertaining to or affecting only one eye.

mononucleosis a blood disease in which the number of monocytes (large, single-nuclear white blood cells) is increased.

mucoid resembling mucus.

mucopurulent containing mucus and pus.

mucosa a mucous membrane.

mucoviscidosis a condition characterized by accumulation of very thick tenacious mucus in the important mucus-secreting glands, involving especially the pancreas.

mural pertaining to the wall of a cavity, organ, or vessel.

murmur an abnormal, soft, blowing sound, not necessarily significant.

myalgia muscular pain.

myasthenia muscular weakness.

mydriasis abnormal dilatation of the pupils of the eye.

mydriatic a drug that dilates the pupils.

myelogram x-ray visualization of the spinal cord after the injection of a radiopaque substance.

myocardium the muscular wall of the heart.

myringotomy incision of the ear drum.

narcolepsy an irresistible tendency to attacks of deep sleep, especially in the daytime.

nausea sensation of discomfort or distress in the area of the stomach.

necrosis localized death of tissue.

necrotic refers to death of a cell or group of cells as a result of injury or disease.

necrotizing causing necrosis.

neoplasm an abnormal new growth of cells or tissue that serves no useful purpose; a tumor.

nephritis any one of a group of conditions in which there is inflammation of the kidney.

nephropathy kidney disease.

nephrosclerosis hardening of the kidney.

nephrosis any degenerative but not inflammatory condition of the kidney.

neuralgia severe, paroxysmal pain along the course of one or more nerves.

neurologist a specialist in the treatment of nervous system disorders.

neuropathy disease of some part of the nervous system.

neuropsychiatric referring to a condition that is both neurological and psychiatric in character.

neurotropic having an affinity for the nervous system.

nevus a small lesion of the skin; may be flat or elevated, pigmented or not, with or without the growth of hair; also called a mole.

nocturia excessive urination during the night.

nocturnal nightly, or occurring at night.

nodule a small protuberance, knob, or swelling.

nucleus pulposus the pulpy mass in the center of an intervertebral disc.

nyctalopia inability to see in dim light; night blindness.

nystagmus involuntary, jerky, repetitive movements of the eyeballs.

obesity fatness.

obstetrician a physician who specializes in the care of women in childbirth.

obturator any structure that occludes an opening.

occipital   pertaining to the back part of the head (the occiput).

occult   detectable only by chemical or microscopic means.

oculomotor   pertaining to movements of the eyeball.

oligomenorrhea   abnormally infrequent or scanty menstruation.

oliguria   deficient secretion of urine in relation to the amount of fluid intake.

ophthalmologist   a physician who specializes in the diseases and refractive errors of the eyes.

opisthotonus   position of extreme extension of the body in which only the head and the heels rest on the surface of the bed.

optician   a person who makes and adjusts eyeglasses and optical instruments.

optometrist   a person trained to examine eyes and prescribe eyeglasses.

organism   a living cell or group of cells; any living individual, either plant or animal.

oronasal   pertaining to the mouth and nose.

orthopedist   a physician who specializes in the treatment of diseases of the musculoskeletal system.

orthopnea   inability to breathe except in an upright, sitting position.

orthostatic   pertains to a condition caused by standing erect.

osteoarthritis   chronic, degenerative arthritis.

osteoarthropy   a disorder of the bones and joints characterized by severe pain and clubbing of the fingers.

osteoblast   a bone-forming cell.

osteomyelitis   inflammation of a bone caused by a pus-forming bacterium.

otitis media   inflammation of the middle ear, characterized by pain, fever, bulging of the eardrum, and ringing sounds.

otologist   a physician specializing in the diseases of the ear.

otoscopy   examination of the external ear canal with a lighted instrument (otoscope).

ovariectomy   removal of one or both ovaries.

pacemaker   (1) the sinoatrial node in the heart; (2) electric pacemaker: a device that can substitute for a defective natural pacemaker.

palliative   providing relief but not curing.

pallor   paleness.

palpable   capable of being felt.

palpation   the act of feeling with the hands.

palpebral fissure   the opening between the two eyelids.

palpitation   rapid heartbeat that is felt by the patient.

Papanicolaou smear   a slide prepared for microscopic study of cells from various body secretions (especially from the genitourinary tract) to detect the presence of a malignant process.

papilledema   edema of the optic disc (at the back of the eyeball); indicative of intracranial pressure.

papular   refers to a papule.

papule   a small, solid, usually round or conical, circumscribed elevation on the skin.

paranasal   near the nasal cavities.

paranoia   a chronic, slowly progressive psychiatric disorder characterized by delusions of grandeur or of persecution; **paranoid** and **paranoidal** are the adjectives.

paraplegia   paralysis of the lower half of the body.

parenchyma   the specialized tissue of an organ; is concerned with its function.

paresis   slight or partial paralysis.

paresthesia   abnormal touch sensation such as burning, tingling, creeping, or pricking.

parotitis   infection of one or both parotid glands; mumps.

paroxysmal   coming on in attacks or spasms.

passive exercises   exercises performed by a therapist, the patient being relaxed.

pathological fracture   a fracture caused by local disease of the bone; also called **spontaneous fracture**.

pathology   the medical science that deals with the cause and nature of disease and the changes that result from disease processes.

pediatrician   a physician who specializes in the problems and diseases of young children.

pellagra   a deficiency disease caused by lack of vitamin B complex in the diet.

pendulous   hanging down.

peptic   pertaining to the stomach.

percussion   a diagnostic procedure consisting of tapping or striking the body.

perforation   a hole in an intact sheet of tissue; may be pathogenic or intentional in nature.

perfusion   the act of spreading over or through, specifically the artificial passage of fluid through an organ or tissue by way of the blood vessels.

pericarditis   inflammation of the outer covering of the heart.

pericranium   the periosteum (covering of the bone) of the skull.

perineum   the area between the vulva and the anus in the female and between the scrotum and the anus in the male.

periorbital   pertaining to the periosteum of the eye socket.

periosteum   the thick, fibrous membrane that covers bones, except at the joints.

peripheral   pertaining to or situated near the outer surface of the body, or to the parts away from the center of the body.

peripheral vascular disease   disorder of the circulation, particularly in the extremities.

peristalsis   wavelike movement of the intestine and certain other structures that are tubular in shape; the motion propels the contents of the lumen forward.

peritoneum   the smooth, delicate membrane that lines the abdominal and pelvic cavities and also covers the organs within them.

pertussis   whooping cough.

pessary   a device inserted into the vagina to support the uterus.

petechia   a pinpoint hemorrhage into the skin.

pharmacotherapy   treatment with drugs.

pharynx   the upper expanded part of the digestive tube that forms the cavity at the back of the mouth.

phenomenon   an unusual occurrence or fact.

phlebitis   inflammation of a vein.

phlebotomy   the act of opening a vein for the purpose of letting blood.

photophobia   inability to expose the eyes to light, or the dread of light.

physiatrist   a physician who specializes in the use of such physical agents as light, heat, water, electricity, and mechanical apparatus.

pigmentation   the deposit of pigment in any body tissue, especially the skin.

pituitary   a small endocrine gland located in the sphenoid bone of the skull; it secretes several hormones that have an effect on other endocrine glands.

plaque   a patch or flat area; an **atheromatous plaque** is a deposit of predominantly fatty material in the lining of a blood vessel.

plethoric   full, overloaded.

pleura   the serous membrane that envelops the lung and lines the chest cavity.

pleurisy   inflammation of the covering of the lung (**pleura**); adjective is **pleuritic**.

pneumoconiosis   dust disease, caused by long continued inhalation of dust in industrial occupations such as coal mining or stone cutting.

pneumoencephalogram   an x-ray picture of the brain after replacement of the cerebrospinal fluid with air or a gas.

pneumothorax   air or gas in the pleural cavity, that is, the potential space between the covering of the lungs and the lining of the chest cavity.

polydipsia   frequent drinking because of excessive thirst.

polyneuropathy   a disease condition in which several nerves are affected.

polyopia   seeing several images of a single object.

polyp   a small, smooth fingerlike growth arising from a mucous surface.

polyphagia   excessive eating or excessive appetite.

polysaccharide   a carbohydrate that when broken down yields ten or more monosaccharides (simple sugars that cannot be broken down any further).

polyuria   the excretion of an excessive amount of urine.

postural drainage   drainage that is achieved by putting the patient in a position in which gravity aids the process.

precordial   pertaining to the region over the heart and stomach.

premonitory   giving advance warning or notice.

presbycusis   impairment of hearing due to aging.

proctologist   a physician who specializes in diseases of the rectum.

proctoscopy   examination of the rectum and lower part of the intestine with a specially designed instrument (**proctoscope**).

prodromal   preceding; said of the period preceding the clinical onset of a disease.

prognosis   a forecast of the probable course, duration, and outcome of a disease.

prolapse   the falling down or downward displacement of an organ or part.

proliferating   increasing in size by cell division.

proprioceptive   refers to the nerve endings in the deeper structures of the body, which are responsible for the sensation of the position of the body in space.

prostration   complete exhaustion.

prothrombin time a test to determine the deficiency in the blood of clotting factors I, II, VII, and X.

pruritus itching of the skin, commonly due to allergies, infestation by parasites, or skin disorders; may be subjective without apparent cause.

psychic pertaining to the mind.

psychogenic originating in the mind.

psychomotor pertaining to the motor effect of the brain or psychic activity.

psychosis a severe mental disorder that arises in the mind.

psychosomatic usually refers to an illness that can be traced to an emotional cause.

psychotherapeutic pertaining to the effect of therapy that utilizes psychological methods.

psychotherapy a form of treatment based on psychological methods rather than on medical, surgical, or pharmacological methods.

psychotropic pertaining to drugs or agents that exert an influence on the mind.

ptosis a drooping, falling, or sinking down of an organ or part.

pulmonary pertaining to the lungs.

pulse deficit the difference in the rate of the heartbeat counted by stethoscope and at the wrist.

punch biopsy the removal of tissue (for examination) by a special instrument called a punch.

purine a protein constituent from which uric acid is derived.

purulent pertaining to, resembling, containing, or producing pus.

pustule a circumscribed raised area on the skin that contains pus.

pyelitis inflammation of the pelvis of the kidney.

pyelogram an x-ray of the renal pelvis and ureter.

pyelonephritis a type of kidney infection that spreads outward from the pelvis of the kidney to the cortex.

pyelonephrosis any disease of the pelvis of the kidney.

pyogenic pus-forming.

quadrant for descriptive purposes, anatomical areas that are roughly circular are divided into four areas called **quadrants**; the abdominal area is divided into right and left, upper and lower quadrants.

quadriplegia paralysis of both arms and both legs.

radicle one of the smallest branches of a nerve or blood vessel.

radicular pertaining to a root or a rootlike structure (see **radicle**).

radioactive having the property of giving off rays due to the spontaneous breaking up of atoms.

radiologist a specialist in the use of x-rays and other forms of radiant energy.

rales abnormal sounds heard in the lungs when fluid is present in the bronchi.

rational of sound mind, not delirious.

rectobulbar (1) behind the eyeball; (2) behind the medulla oblongata.

rectocele protrusion of part of the rectum through the wall of the vagina; caused by injury to the posterior vaginal wall.

reduce to restore something to its usual place, as in hernia, dislocation, or fracture.

regurgitation backward flow, as of stomach contents into the mouth or of blood between the chambers of the heart when the valves do not function properly.

remission a period of lessening or abatement of the symptoms of a disease.

renal pertaining to the kidney.

replacement therapy the giving of a glandular substance or hormone to compensate for the absence or deficiency of the particular substance in the body.

retinitis inflammation of the retina, the delicate innermost coat of the eye.

retinopathy any inflammatory condition of the retina.

retrograde going backward.

rotating tourniquets a system of treatment in which tourniquets are applied to all four extremities in turn, as near the trunk as possible; one is released every 10 or 15 minutes, so that three are always in place.

sarcoid a tumor resembling a sarcoma.

sarcoma a tumor that arises in the connective tissue; often highly malignant.

scapula the shoulder blade.

sclerosis abnormal hardening of a tissue.

scoliosis lateral curvature of the spine.

scotoma an area of darkness or blindness within the field of vision.

sebaceous glands small glands in the skin that secrete an oily, colorless substance through the hair follicles.

seborrhea   a greasy condition of the skin of the face, scalp, and elsewhere, usually accompanied by itching and burning; due to overactivity of the sebaceous glands of the skin.

secondary infection   an infection that is imposed on another infection.

sedative   a drug or agent that reduces physical activity.

sedimentation rate   the rate at which blood cells settle to the bottom of a tube of drawn blood; differs in different diseases and in different stages of a disease; abbreviated **ESR** and **sed. rate**.

seizure   (1) a sudden attack such as a convulsion; (2) an epileptic fit.

self-limiting   running a definite course regardless of external factors or influences.

senile   pertaining to old age; usually refers to mental deterioration whether or not accompanied by physical deterioration.

septum   a thin partition between two cavities.

shock   a serious state in which body processes are profoundly reduced as a result of injury, severe illness, or circulatory disturbance; features include low blood pressure, pallor, rapid pulse, restlessness, thirst, cold and clammy skin.

sicca   dry.

sinoatrial node   a small mass of specialized cells in the upper part of the right atrium where the electrical impulses of the heart originate; also called **S-A node**.

sinus   a hollow or cavity, especially one in a bone of the cranium.

sinusitis   inflammation of one or more sinuses.

sloughing   the formation of a mass of necrotic tissue that separates from the healthy tissue and is eventually washed away by exudated serum.

smegma   a foul-smelling secretion that accumulates in the folds of the vagina and under the prepuce of the penis.

specific gravity   the weight of a substance as compared with an equal volume of water.

sphincter   a circular muscle that contracts to narrow a natural passage or close a natural opening in the body.

splenomegaly   enlargement of the spleen.

sputum   excess saliva and secretion from the respiratory passages, expectorated through the mouth.

staphylococcus   a genus of bacteria, spherical in shape and tending to occur in grapelike clusters.

stasis   stagnation or stoppage of flow of blood, urine, or other body fluid, or of the motion of a part.

steatorrhea   a syndrome due to various defects of absorption from the intestine; stools are bulky, pale, and greasy.

stenosis   abnormal narrowing of any canal or orifice.

sternum   the breastbone.

stertorous   breathing that is characterized by snoring.

stethoscope   an instrument for listening to various body sounds such as the heartbeat.

stomatitis   inflammation of the mucous membranes of the mouth.

streptococcus   a genus of bacteria, spherical in shape, usually occurring in chains of varying length.

stricture   an abnormal narrowing of a tubular structure.

stridor   a harsh, high-pitched sound in breathing, caused by air passing through constricted air passages.

subclinical   the period in the course of a disease when the symptoms are not severe enough to make the disease identifiable.

subcutaneous   beneath the skin.

sublingual   beneath the tongue.

subperiostal   beneath the periosteum.

substernal   beneath the sternum.

substitution therapy   see replacement therapy.

subxiphoid   below the lower part of the sternum.

superior vena cava   the large vein that collects the blood from the head, chest, and arms and returns it to the heart.

superior vena cava syndrome   obstruction of the superior vena cava by tumor or other condition; causes edema and enlargement of the blood vessels of the face, neck, and arms, as well as coughing and difficult breathing.

suppuration   the formation of pus.

suprapubic   above the pubic bone.

symmetrical   refers to the condition when corresponding parts of the body are of the same shape, size, and general characteristics.

sympathectomy   surgical removal of a sympathetic nerve or interruption of sympathetic nerve pathways.

sympathomimetic   simulation of autonomic nerve action.

syncope   fainting.

syndrome   a group of symptoms or signs that, occurring together, produce a pattern that is characteristic of a particular disease or disorder.

synovial fluid   fluid secreted by the membrane lining joint cavities; its function is lubrication to minimize friction during joint movement.

syringomyelia   an uncommon progressive disease of the nervous system, characterized by interference with the sensation of pain and temperature so that injuries such as burns are painless.

systole the period of contraction of the heart muscle in the heartbeat.

tabes dorsalis a variety of syphilis of the nervous system, characterized by muscular incoordination, ataxia, joint disorders, neuralgia, and sometimes paralysis.

tachycardia excessively rapid action of the heart with resulting increase in the pulse rate.

tactile pertaining to the sense of touch.

tendon reflex the contraction of a muscle when the tendon attached to it is tapped; for example, the knee jerk reflex when the leg just below the knee cap is tapped.

tenesmus painful, ineffectual straining to empty the bladder or rectum.

testosterone the male hormone, secreted in the testes.

thromboangiitis obliterans an uncommon vascular disorder of unknown cause that occurs chiefly in young males, characterized by pain in the calf of the leg; also called **Buerger's disease.**

thrombophlebitis inflammation of the wall of a vein with formation of a thrombus.

thrombosis the formation or presence of a blood clot within a blood vessel.

thrombus a clot formed by coagulation of blood in a blood vessel; remains in the location in which it was formed.

thyrotoxicosis a toxic condition due to excessive production of the thyroid gland hormone (thyroxine), characterized by anxiety, rapid heartbeat, weight loss, and later, prominence of the eyeballs.

tinnitus subjective noises such as ringing, roaring, or humming that accompany certain hearing disorders.

tonic a state of continuous contraction, said of muscles.

tonometry the measurement of pressure; often refers to intraocular pressure.

tophi small, hard formations in the earlobes or certain other tissues.

toxic poisonous.

trachea the windpipe.

tracheostomy the surgical creation of an opening into the trachea through the front of the neck.

traction a steady drawing or pulling exerted by hand or with a mechanical device, used in the treatment of fractures and various other pathologic conditions or deformities.

tranquilizer   a drug or agent that acts by reducing tension and anxiety.

transfusion   the introduction of a fluid, usually blood, directly into the bloodstream.

trauma   a wound or injury caused by external force or violence.

tremor   involuntary trembling or quivering.

tubercle   (1) a small rounded elevation or nodule on the skin; (2) a small rounded eminence on a bone; (3) the specific lesion in tuberculosis.

tumor   a swelling or enlargement due to pathological overgrowth of tissue.

tunica vaginalis   the serous sheath that covers the testes and epididymis.

turbid   opaque or cloudy.

turbinate bones   scroll-shaped bones on either side of the lateral nasal walls.

tympanic membrane   the eardrum.

ulcer   an open, circumscribed lesion on the surface of the skin or of a membrane.

umbilical   refers to the umbilicus, the scar or pit in the center of the abdominal wall left by the separation of the umbilical cord after birth.

unilateral   involving only one side of a structure or of the body.

urates   salts of uric acid; sodium urate is found in the stony or gritty deposits that accumulate in the tissues around the joints in gout.

uremia   a serious condition in which kidney failure results in retention of nitrogenous substances in the blood.

urinalysis   examination of the urine by laboratory methods.

urologist   a physician who specializes in the diseases of the urinary system.

urticaria   hives.

varices   dilated, tortuous blood vessels, particularly veins; varicose veins.

varicose veins   veins that are swollen or distended, especially in the legs.

varicosity   a varicose vein.

vascular   related to or referring to blood vessels.

vasodilator   (1) certain nerves of the involuntary nervous system that cause the muscles of arterial walls to relax with a consequent lowering of blood pressure; (2) agents that cause dilatation of the arterioles and consequent lowering of blood pressure.

vasopressin   the antidiuretic hormone.

venous stasis   a stoppage or slackening of blood flow in the veins.

vertigo   a sensation of whirling, either of one's self or of the world around one.

vesicle   a small, elevated, circumscribed, fluid-containing lesion on the skin; a blister.

virus   a microorganism that cannot be seen with an ordinary microscope but is capable of producing disease.

visceral   pertaining to internal organs, especially those of the trunk.

vital capacity   the amount of air that can be expelled from the lungs after a deep breath.

xanthelasma   formation of yellowish spots or plaques on the eyelids.

xanthochromia   yellowish discoloration, usually of the skin.

Index

Date